Primary Care Ethics

Edited by

Deborah Bowman
Senior Lecturer in Medical Ethics and Law
St George's, University of London

and

John Spicer
General Practitioner, South London
Associate Director in GP Education
London Deanery, University of London

Foreword by

Roger Higgs
Professor Emeritus in General Practice and Primary Care
King's College London

Radcliffe Publishing
Oxford • New York

Radcliffe Publishing Ltd
18 Marcham Road
Abingdon
Oxon OX14 1AA
United Kingdom

www.radcliffe-oxford.com
Electronic catalogue and worldwide online ordering facility.

British Library Cataloguing in Publication Data

A catalogue record for this book is available from the British Library.

ISBN-10: 1 85775 730 0
ISBN-13: 978 1 85775 730 9

Typeset by Lapiz Digital Services, Chennai, India
Printed and bound by TJI Digital, Padstow, Cornwall, UK

Contents

Foreword

You have opened this book. Whether you buy it or borrow it, I know you should read it.

Why am I so sure? You have shown you are involved in or interested in primary medical care or ethics, maybe both. To echo what Paul Freeling once said about research in primary care, I could say, 'Show me a consultation and I'll show you an ethical issue'. This claim makes sense in part because medicine is at base a moral enterprise: although it has been professionalised, it owes its existence to the strong moral force that most of us feel, to help the sick and suffering. But that urge to help may face challenges. On a broad perspective, moral concerns may have to hold their own against competing arguments coming from other sources like economics or politics. At the other end of the scale, when an individual clinician feels 'stuck' in an encounter with a patient and doesn't know what to do, the decision crisis seldom centres round factual issues like the dose of a drug, but concerns the sorts of questions that at once take us into the moral arena. Should I tell this person what's really wrong? What should I do when they are pressing me to do something I don't think I should do? Is this really my job? Who is responsible for sorting out this mess? Why do I feel so angry in this situation? My own gloss on the original claim could now be, 'Show me as well a strong emotion in primary care and I'll show you an ethical issue', but whether you agree with me or not, we can be sure that the answers to most problematic encounters will not be found in the *BNF*.

This is not a moral cookbook, however, so most of those sort of problems won't be 'solved' by reading these essays: but the reader will be helped to begin to make the journey out of the maze by what she or he finds here. The emphasis is different too from other writing in medical ethics, where much of the focus is on frontier scientific issues. Important as these are in all sectors of the health service, the major moral questions that interest these authors (and interested Alastair Campbell and me when we wrote *In That Case* back in 1982) lie elsewhere, at the interface between patients' lives, their hopes and values, and the possible responses of professionals working in structures that are not necessarily of their own choosing. These questions, then, are not posed out at the unfrequented frontiers but in the everyday experience of life as everyone lives it. Issues of blame, complexity, choice, rights, care, competence, boundaries, motivation, working together — all these and many other concepts frame and form the work of primary care. Whether you are young and just starting, facing an exam, bored and not sure why, distressed, euphoric or just plain overworked, you should read what these experienced writers say. Neither you nor 'it' — whatever that is — will be quite the same again, I can promise.

Roger Higgs MBE, MA, MB, FRCP, FRCGP
January 2007

About the editors

Deborah Bowman is a Senior Lecturer in Medical Ethics and Law at St George's, University of London and leads the Personal and Professional Development Theme for the Graduate Entry Programme. She has previously worked for Queen Mary and Westfield College and The Open University. She acts as Honorary Secretary to the St George's NHS Trust Clinical Ethics Forum. Her particular research interests are medical error and accountability in primary care, confidentiality and education in ethics.

John Spicer is a GP in South London and a Clinical Tutor in Medical Law and Ethics at St George's, University of London. He has interests in medical humanities and the nature of personal responsibility in health. He is interested in educational process and teaches on several courses in education for the London Deanery, where he is an Associate Director in GP postgraduate education.

List of contributors

Andrew Dicker has been an inner-city GP in London since 1991. He is a GP trainer and course organiser for the Bloomsbury/Royal Free & UCH Vocational Training Scheme. He has also been involved in undergraduate teaching for several years and is an honorary Senior Clinical Lecturer at Imperial College.

Ann King is a health visitor working in Croydon Primary Care Trust. She has a diploma in medical ethics and she also works as a clinical ethicist within the PCT. Ann is a guest lecturer on several undergraduate and postgraduate programmes at St George's, University of London.

Margaret Lloyd is Professor of Primary Care and Medical Education at the Royal Free and University College Medical School, London. She is Vice Dean (Curriculum) and leads the Professional Development Spine, which is one of the vertical components of the new undergraduate curriculum. She is also a part-time general practitioner in north London.

Michael Parker is Professor of Bioethics at the University of Oxford and Director of the Ethox Centre. The Ethox Centre is a multidisciplinary research centre bringing together sociologists, anthropologists, philosophers, lawyers and clinicians to carry out research on the ethical, social and legal implications of developments in medical science and practice. Michael is also Honorary Clinical Ethicist at the Oxford Radcliffe Hospitals Trust providing ethics support in the clinical setting and to medical researchers and is a member of several national committees including: the ethics committee of the Royal College of Physicians, and the steering committee of the UK Clinical Ethics Network committee. With Angus Clarke and Anneke Lucassen, he also runs the UK Genethics Club (www.genethicsclub.org).

Henk Parmentier works as a GP with a special interest in mental health in London and was trained at the University of Utrecht, the Netherlands. He is a member of the South London Primary Care Network (STaRNet), facilitating and conducting primary care research. He is a trustee of Primary Care Mental Health & Education (PriMHE). He has served on the Croydon LREC and was attached as a physician to the continuing care unit of the Croydon Old Age Psychiatrists.

Jim Price trained in general medicine whilst serving in the Royal Navy in the 1980s. In 1990, he left the navy and since then has been a GP in

Chichester. He is an experienced GP trainer as well as GP tutor for the local area. Since 2001, he has been a part-time Senior Lecturer in Primary Care at the University of Brighton, and is now Programme Leader for Professional Development at the Postgraduate Medical School. He has also been involved with the development of the clinical curriculum at the Brighton and Sussex Medical School, and has a particular interest in the teaching of professionalism and ethics. His research interests are influenced by complexity science and its relationship to clinical leadership, health professional education, organisational development and health services management.

Anne Slowther is Senior Lecturer in Clinical Ethics at Warwick Medical School. She runs the undergraduate and postgraduate ethics teaching courses, and conducts research on ethical decision-making in primary care. She is also a visiting Fellow at the Ethox Centre, University of Oxford where she oversees the National Clinical Ethics Network support programme and takes the lead within the Centre on the development and delivery of individual ethics support for clinicians and other healthcare providers. She began her work in clinical ethics in 1999 and prior to this was a full-time GP in Manchester. She is a member of the *Journal of Medical Ethics* Advisory Committee and a member of the Editorial Board of the recently launched *Clinical Ethics Journal*.

Peter D Toon is a GP in East Kent and Director of Postgraduate Education and Development in the Centre for Health Sciences at Queen Mary School of Medicine, University of London. He has been interested in the philosophical basis of general practice for many years and has published a number of papers on the subject, most notably RCGP Occasional Papers 65 and 74, which taken together lay out a vision of good medical practice that emphasises the importance of personal qualities the practitioner needs to flourish as a GP – qualities often called virtues. He is currently engaged in further work on the characterisation of the virtuous practitioner.

Katharine Wright was based for nine years in the research service of the House of Commons Library, advising MPs of all parties on healthcare law and policy. After completing a Masters in medical law and ethics at King's College London in 1999, she was seconded to the Department of Health to work on consent to treatment issues. She is now based at the NHS Litigation Authority, providing information to the NHS on the impact of the Human Rights Act on healthcare law.

Paquita de Zulueta is a part-time GP in West London and Honorary Senior Clinical Lecturer at Imperial College. She has been involved in postgraduate general practice education since 2003 and is currently involved in the educational supervision of PRHOs in the practice. She provides teaching for the Medical Ethics MSc at Imperial College, and has taught medical ethics and law to undergraduates and postgraduates since 2003. She is chair of the Health Care Ethics Forum and has been a member of research ethics and clinical ethics committees for several years. She has written papers and undertaken research on antenatal HIV testing and role models in undergraduate medicine. She also has an interest in medicine and literature and facilitates a reading group for GPs and other professionals.

Acknowledgements

'Acknowledge' seems like a rather inadequate word to describe the gratitude we feel towards those who have unfailingly supported us through this project. However, knowing that those same supporters would dislike a gushing expression of thanks, acknowledge these important people is what we shall do.

Wittgenstein reminds us that 'knowledge is, in the end, based on acknowledgement' and in the case of the knowledge, ideas and arguments advanced in this volume, this assertion could not be more accurate. First, as editors, we would like to acknowledge the hard work, creativity and commitment of our contributors. Without their individual passion for particular subjects and universal ability to make their areas of special interest accessible and engaging, this collection would simply not exist. Their patience with a somewhat flexible time scale and prompt responses to our persistent intrusions into their already busy working lives made our job far easier than it may otherwise have been. Gillian Nineham and Lisa Abbott at Radcliffe have supported this project from the outset. Their encouragement, professionalism and efficiency ensured that the vague ideas we first took to Gillian developed into this book.

To the staff and students at St George's and colleagues in the primary care clinics of South West London, we would like to express our sincere thanks. The thought-provoking questions from, and perspectives of, students in teaching sessions and the serendipitous coffee room discussions with colleagues have been more influential than they probably realise. Finally, although the cover of this book suggests that there are two editors, we believe that there has been an editorial team. There are some important members of that team who have neither official contributor nor editor status, but whose support, love and help has been immeasurably important, not merely in this project, but in our lives — our families.

Introduction

The market for books about healthcare ethics is increasingly crowded. There are options for every kind of reader, from those choosing to reflect on healthcare ethics at doctoral level, to those encountering ethics for the first time as a required element of demanding undergraduate training. So why another book, and what does this title have to offer readers whose shelves may already be groaning under the weight of volumes containing the word 'ethics' in their titles?

The idea, as originally conceived, was that this text would offer thought-provoking, but selective, perspectives on primary care ethics for readers who were seeking material that moved beyond the 'entry level' texts. That we chose primary care as the healthcare context for the project is partly borne out of the editors' clinical and research interests, and partly a consequence of our belief that primary care presents different ethical questions for healthcare professionals. It is much more than merely a location. The 'tertiary' level ethical problems that dominate so much of the debate about healthcare ethics, such as genetics, cloning, organ donation and research, are experienced entirely differently in primary care. Moreover, what might be argued to be core moral principles, such as autonomy and justice, may be reinterpreted when viewed through the lens of primary care. The unique flavour of primary healthcare is familiar to all our contributors and we believe their familiarity with the particular context of primary care has resulted in some thought-provoking and novel accounts of even well-rehearsed moral debates.

This collection does not claim to be a definitive and comprehensive guide to all the ethical questions that might arise in primary care. The selection of themes for inclusion was 'bottom up' in that we approached contributors whom we believe have interesting and original perspectives on ethics in primary care, and encouraged them to pursue areas of particular interest. The result of this approach is that the book covers a wide and eclectic range of themes. The word 'theme' is important: this is not a topic-based volume in which the reader is led through 'birth to death issues'. Rather, the chapters describe concepts, theories and constructs that may be relevant, no matter what the clinical issue or the type of patient; for example, we seek to stimulate thought and discussion on themes such as truth, trust, virtue, accountability, clinical ethics education, professional identities, rights and complexity theory.

It is this theme-based approach to ethical discussion and analysis, in conjunction with the primary care focus, that we believe makes this text worthy of a place on groaning bookshelves. Those who decide to make space in their study or office will, we hope, be rewarded with varied, stimulating and original contributions to their understanding of primary care ethics. Each chapter can be read as a discrete essay. However, we have tried to ensure a narrative logic in the chronology of the chapters and to include explicit cross-references where we believe one contributor's ideas inform another's submission. Broadly speaking, the first half of the book is concerned with the relationships between healthcare professionals and patients. In contrast, the second half of the book reflects on professional values and intra-professional ethics.

In Chapter 1, Paquita de Zulueta examines the cornerstone of the therapeutic relationship and discusses truth and trust in a changing world of healthcare. The therapeutic relationship is discussed further by Margaret Lloyd in Chapter 2, where she analyses autonomy in relation to primary care. The relationship between choice and responsibility is explored by John Spicer in Chapter 3, followed by Katharine Wright's discussion in Chapter 4 of the application of rights theory to primary care. In Chapter 5, Henk Parmentier, John Spicer and Ann King examine the challenges of care where a patient lacks capacity to decide for him or herself. Chapter 6 is the bridging chapter in the book: Peter Toon discusses virtue theory in relation to primary care and what it offers to primary care practitioners, both in how they work with patients and each other. Ann King picks up the theme of working relationships from the interprofessional perspective in Chapter 7, reflecting both on the value of multidisciplinary teamworking and its challenges. In Chapter 8, Jim Price and Deborah Bowman analyse complexity theory and how it might inform professional ethics in primary care. Chapter 9 consists of a powerfully articulated piece by Andrew Dicker arguing that doctors (and he explains why he has limited his analysis to doctors) have a moral duty to care for themselves as well as their patients. In Chapter 10, Deborah Bowman discusses recent changes in professional accountability and the vexed issue of the under-performing healthcare professional, with particular reference to the use of discretion and judgment. Finally, Anne Slowther and Mike Parker describe the growth of clinical ethics support in the UK, and the potential value to primary care of such support. As editors, we draw the volume to a close with our reflections on the project and some cautious crystal-ball gazing about the themes we believe may direct future discussions of ethics in primary care.

Finally, a word about the claims of this book to serve primary care rather than solely general practice. All our contributors have sought to offer inclusive analyses or explain their reasoning for focusing on one professional group. However, we believe that the development of a truly cross-professional ethic of primary care is one of the greatest challenges facing all healthcare professionals. We were struck repeatedly by the paucity of interprofessional literature on ethics in relation to most, if not all, of the chapters. Uniprofessional perspectives are common place, but a shared analysis is a rare bird in the ethical literature. Given the increasing (and, we believe, welcome) emphasis on interprofessional teams in primary care, we would be gratified if this project allows multiprofessional groups to discuss some of the themes contained and contributes here to the development of a truly integrated ethic of primary healthcare.

Deborah Bowman and John Spicer
January 2007

Chapter 1

Truth, trust and the doctor–patient relationship

Paquita de Zulueta

> It is trite to describe the health professional's relationship with his or her patient as a relationship of trust, yet the description encapsulates the very heart of the relationship.
>
> Margaret Brazier and Mary Lobjoit[1]

Introduction

'Trust' is such a small word, yet it holds such significance. But what *is* trust? It eludes definition, yet, instinctively, most of us have a clear sense of what it is, and, in particular, when it is lacking. We know and value its importance – indeed necessity – in everyday life, as in medicine, but we may have difficulty articulating precisely why. We notice it much as we notice air – only when it becomes scarce or polluted.

Trust has been described as 'the truly mysterious, barely known entity that holds society and ourselves together, the "dark matter" of the soul'[2] or as 'the God particle [...] the fuel, the essence, the foundation of general practice'.[3] The *Oxford Shorter Dictionary* defines 'to trust' as 'to have faith or confidence in; to rely on or depend upon' – a definition that fails to capture the complexity and richness of the concept.

I shall be examining the extent to which trust underpins the doctor–patient relationship; what promotes trust and what undermines it in this context. I shall focus on the relevance of truthfulness in the promotion of trust between patients and their GPs. My further aim is to clarify the philosophical foundations for the variety of models representing the doctor–patient relationship and to choose the one that best encompasses and fosters trust. I shall not be examining the metaphysics of truth, albeit a subject of great interest and recently explored by two modern philosophers, Bernard Williams[4] and Simon Blackburn.[5] I am aware that by narrowing the scope of the enquiry, I will omit issues relevant to trust – a multi-faceted phenomenon – yet hope that the enquiry will nevertheless yield fruitful insights.

If we stop to consider how people would function in the absence of trust, we soon realise that ordinary life would be impossible. We regularly put our trust in others (and machines made by others) when we undertake banal activities such as driving a car, asking for directions, drawing money from a cash point, posting a letter, confiding in a friend, having our hair cut or buying books from an Internet-based retailer such as Amazon. Trust pervades our daily life and gives us a degree of predictability and confidence. In the end, we have to place our trust in others to engage with the world. Without trust we are doomed to self-imprisonment.

Those who break our trust, not only betray us, but threaten the very fabric of civilised society. In Dante's *Inferno,* traitors went directly to the innermost circle of Hell, closest to Satan himself. As O'Hara says:

> Perhaps Dante's instincts are sounder than ours: perhaps those who betray trust *are* doing serious and dangerous violence to the foundations of society. Minor betrayals, individually less shocking than the crimes we see in our newspaper headlines, make us less capable of getting on with each other, of living the lives we want to lead.[6]

Ruth Etchells also argues that a culture that accepts 'personal perfidy' – the acceptance of breaches of trust – generates mistrust and cynicism about professional and public matters nowadays, as it did in Elizabethan times.[7] And yet, as Annette Baier reminds us, trust is neutral, and 'exploitation and conspiracy, as much as justice and fellowship, thrive better in an atmosphere of trust'.[8]

I shall be focusing on *personal* trust as distinct from *social* trust. Individuals gain personal trust and institutions social trust.[9] To give an example: in present-day Iraq, interpersonal trust may be high between relatives or a tribal group, but social trust low for the institutions governing law and order. To give another example, trust in a doctor may be high, but low for the NHS generally. The distinction has been discussed and refined by several sociologists, including Niklas Luhmann, who distinguishes between trust in persons and confidence in institutions.[10] Trust in persons requires the ontological freedom of the other – it becomes 'the generalised expectation that the other will handle his freedom, his disturbing potential for diverse action, in keeping with his personality – or, rather with the personality which he has presented and made socially visible'.[11]

Both forms of trust are necessary to reduce complexity and keep chaos at bay. To trust is to venture into the unknown. Confidence (or reliance), in contrast, is based on past performance, the ability to impose sanctions in case of 'betrayal' and the power to check up on the actions of the other in the future.[12] The current regulatory frameworks evidently are attempts to increase confidence, but may not necessarily increase trust.

The context

Trust dominates the news and politics. Arguably, the word has been degraded by overuse in recent times. Following the invasion of Iraq by American and allied forces in March 2002, the English media have referred to trust and its betrayal on countless occasions. The Hutton Inquiry[13] revealed an anatomy of deceit. Those under scrutiny provided a broad palette of every shade of deception: from evasion to concealment, to partial disclosure, to deliberate non-disclosure, and thence to sophistry, half truths, distortions, and, eventually, to frank lies. The Inquiry gave evidence of how people can intentionally mislead others by manipulating facts and theories to suit their own agendas. Albeit not directly relevant to the doctor–patient relationship, Hutton and other allied inquiries provide us with a useful lexicon for dishonesty and deception, and also remind us of the potential for abuse by those in power.

   Medicine in recent times has also experienced a crisis in trust. The discovery that the GP Harold Shipman was a mass murderer and the GP Dr Green a paedophile, the revelation of negligent and arrogant practitioners such as the gynaecologists Rodney Ledward and Richard Neale, and the scandals at hospitals in Bristol and Alder Hey all conjoined to seriously undermine the public's trust in the medical profession. This mistrust was worsened by the discovery that professional self-regulation was found to be seriously deficient and that safeguards to protect vulnerable individuals were insufficient or absent. A number of inquiries followed, resulting in a shake-up of the General Medical Council (GMC), and a (bewildering) number of bodies were set up to monitor and manage clinical performance. In addition, doctors now have compulsory annual appraisal, clinical audit and five-yearly revalidation (the methodology still to be agreed at the time of writing). These changes are discussed in detail in Chapter 10. A new age of accountability is born. And yet, as the philosopher Onora O'Neill reminds us, accountability cannot replace trust. She argues that the new 'accountability culture' creates more administrative control, relentless demands to record and report, detailed conformity to procedures and protocols, and the setting of readily measurable and controllable targets. This culture creates 'perverse incentives', distorts the 'proper aims of professional practice', and undermines institutional autonomy. Slavish adhesion to *extrinsic* incentives – remunerated vaccination targets and 48-hour accessibility are examples of this in general practice – has generated criticism and fuelled mistrust that the medical profession is not pursuing the *intrinsic* requirements of being 'good doctors'. We have the paradox that an increase in accountability may actually reduce and undermine trust.

> The pursuit of ever more perfect accountability provides citizens and consumers, patients and parents with more information, more comparisons, more complaints systems; but it also builds a culture of suspicion, low morale, and may ultimately lead to professional cynicism, and then we would have grounds for public mistrust.[14]

Some would argue that this has already happened. And all that is achieved is that trust is shifted onto other individuals empowered to monitor the professionals – but why should they be any more trustworthy? Meanwhile, the public questions whether doctors are pursuing public health targets and other prescribed ends for the public good or for their own benefit, and doctors question (usually amongst themselves) whether they really are likely to benefit their patients. Choice, not fate, is placed on the shoulders of patients, who have to undertake greater responsibility for failure, of making bad choices. Their only safeguards are those regulatory mechanisms for increasing confidence, and the reliance on the behaviours and attitudes set by socially sanctioned roles.

The relevance of role

How immutable are these socially sanctioned roles and the role of the doctor in particular? In her book, *Rules, Roles and Relations*, Dorothy Emmet defines role as the 'name for a typical relation in which a typical action is expected'.[15] In our roles, we subsume much of our subjectivity, and adopt a persona. But doctors cannot prevent their own personal style or core beliefs from seeping through; otherwise they would conform to fully predictable and uniform patterns of behaviour, which evidence would suggest they clearly do not. Personal and role relationships overlap and the persona cannot be banished from the person or vice versa. Emmet goes on to say that we should not adopt too rigid a view of the persona:

> If we press the 'mask' metaphor and take so mechanical and literal a notion of the *persona* that it becomes just something through which the right sorts of noises sound (*personant*), we shall never catch the conversation-like nuances by which role

performances are also found to be relationships between people.[16]

Seligman suggests that role can be viewed as a stable state within a social system, complete with its normative role expectations, or it can be seen as a process – role-making rather than role-taking – emerging out of interaction and reciprocity, and less determined by systemic constraints. This more fluid and negotiable perception of role allows greater freedom, but less certainty.[17] Patients cannot rely on a bedrock of role predictability from their health professionals. The public's expectations of the GP's role may conflict with that of GPs, creating tensions. Furthermore, GPs may experience role conflict and seek to spend more time with their families whilst pressures mount for them to be available 24/7, even for trivial complaints. Evidence would suggest that young practitioners are more carefully circumscribing their medical role.[18]

A socially or politically sanctioned role may not square with the universal ethics of the profession.[19] If there is a tension between the two, I would argue that doctors should always remain true to the goals of medicine. These, in essence, are to provide the greatest net benefit to their individual patients and to help work towards human flourishing in society at large. These goals must always underpin the physician's role, such that there is an intrinsic and coherent motivation to maintain them. Otherwise doctors are in danger of colluding with inhumane government-led policies such as the euthanasia programme in Nazi Germany[20] or, more recently, the torture of suspected terrorist detainees.[21]

Trust in crisis?

Has the public really lost trust in the profession? Recent opinion polls (bearing in mind that these are also not altogether trustworthy!) still place doctors as the most trusted professionals after nurses, with 90% of those interviewed believing that they could rely on doctors to tell the truth and the same number believing that they are doing their job fairly or very well.[22] *If* trust in medicine and science is declining, paradoxically the reasons for trusting have apparently grown – such as successes in combating diseases, increased efforts to respect persons and their autonomy, and stronger regulations to protect the environment and the performance of doctors. O'Neill concludes that there is not much evidence for a crisis of trust, but more of a 'culture of suspicion', and that the 'crisis' represents: 'an unrealistic hankering for a world in which safety and compliance are total, and breaches of trust are totally eliminated. [...]Trust is needed precisely because all guarantees are incomplete.'[23]

The post-modern condition

If we assume that there *is* a crisis of trust, this may lie not only in the behaviours of renegade professionals, but also in the inherent paradox of the post-modern condition.[24] The enlightenment project has evolved such that the individual has become the final repository for rights and values, the central moral locus of autonomous willed activity. Because of (or despite) globalisation, individuals may experience alienation living in a fragmented and pluralistic world. Identity is no longer a collective attribute, the assumption of shared norms, values and orientations can no longer be assumed, and the idea of a shared moral community is weak. Trust in others relies on familiarity, but, as Seligman says: 'without a shared universe of expectations, histories, memories, or affective commitment, no basis for familiarity can exist'[25] and 'we are forced to rely on trust more and more at the very moment when its presence (and even potential) is receding.'[26]

As trust recedes, we are less able to negotiate our social interactions without hard and fast rules, and this is 'but another manifestation of the replacement of the open-ended negotiation of trust with the rule-bound behaviour of system confidence'.[27] Others present potential danger, and where there is danger, there is the necessity to impose strict legal codes and regulations. Zygmunt Bauman discusses how the popular programmes of *Big Brother*, *Survivor* and *The Weakest Link* convey the message 'trust no one' and epitomise a Darwinian world of survival where trust, compassion and mercy are 'suicidal': 'If you are not tougher and less scrupulous than all the others, you will be done in by them, with or without remorse.'[28]

Alasdair MacIntyre predicted this outcome in his book *After Virtue* and laments the lack of *telos* – the goal of man striving for self-improvement by cultivating the virtues – in contemporary philosophical theories. He argues that the philosophers of the enlightenment (Kant, Hume, Adam Smith and others), by abandoning any idea of *telos* and giving primacy to individual autonomy, gave us an incoherent moral scheme and an unsuccessful project.

> Contemporary moral experience as a consequence has a paradoxical character. For each of us is taught to see himself or herself as an autonomous moral agent; but each of us also becomes engaged by modes of practice, aesthetic or bureaucratic, which involve us in manipulative relationships with one another.[29]

According to MacIntyre, there is no connection between the facts of human nature and the precepts of morality; furthermore these are 'expressly designed to be discrepant with one another'.[30] In this age, solidarity is harder to sustain and self-effacement is eschewed. 'Self-realisation' is the primary goal, with a multiplicity of self-help books and gurus to achieve this, but without a grounding in a shared human endeavour or mutuality. The rise in communitarian philosophies[31] and the resurgence of virtue ethics and the closely related narrative ethics,[32] reflects a counterbalance to the current emphasis on individual autonomy and consumerism. Narrative ethics involves thinking of human life as a narrative unity in a way that is alien to the dominant individualist and bureaucratic modes of modern culture. Readers will find more on virtue ethics and its application to primary care in Chapter 6.

The relevance of information

Redressing this rather gloomy perspective, Richard Horton writes that the new 'information age' (and the advent of the Internet in particular), has redressed the significant information imbalance that used to exist between patients and doctors. Trust, he argues, becomes more circumscribed and relies on a specific technical skill.[33] He acknowledges that a greater public awareness of risk and of the limitations of the expert systems creates an 'institutionalisation of doubt'; yet he views this as liberating for patients and doctors: 'Doctors are wrong to lament loss of trust. Less trust is a good thing, for it suggests transparency regarding the reality of medicine.'[34]

I agree with Horton that doctors need to act more as 'information navigators' rather than 'information givers': together doctor and patient steer through the choppy seas of scientific evidence – some relevant and accurate, some unhelpful or misleading. The doctor acts as the navigator and watchman, marking out the danger zones, whilst at the same time enabling the patient's values and preferences to steer the ship in the direction the patient wants to go. But trust is not based on information alone. Horton himself acknowledges this, and submits that trust is predicated on a belief in the healthcare provider, confidence in the system, dependence on competence working in the system and transcendence from the fear created by ignorance. He does not elaborate on what is meant by these concepts or on their origins. A simple view of the informed patient and doctor encounter could be: a patient has found out that a certain drug is the most effective for his condition and the doctor is willing to prescribe it – end of story. But is this the only possible story? Patients may be confused and anxious even if well informed about their illness. To shoulder this uncertainty alone is a heavy burden for someone who is vulnerable and afraid. John Diamond, in his seminal book, *C: Because cowards get cancer too*, describes these feelings as he scours the Internet:

> I had no way to gauge the relative importance of the words I was reading. Was a paper on neck cancers published in Antwerp in 1992 more or less relevant than one on throat cancers published in Chicago in 1987? Was a trial involving 3,000 patients on chemotherapy as important as one on involving 200 on radiotherapy? I wasn't ready for this yet.[35]

Being given accurate information helps, but cannot provide the entire basis for trust. But perhaps what Horton is really trying to convey is that patients' new-founded scientific literacy encourages them to be more mature and realistic in their expectations, thus liberating doctors. And yet the story does not end here, as Horton recognises. For patients read about 'wonder drugs' and new technologies, and understandably wish to have these to treat their own illnesses. The case of Herceptin (trastuzumab) for breast cancer is a recent example. Lay knowledge is often incomplete and the lay press often distorts the facts, creating misguided optimism.[36] Herceptin is not appropriate for all women with breast cancer and is still under evaluation.[37] But any professional scepticism or caution is viewed as paternalistic or parsimonious. A position of distrust is readily adopted.

The relevance of compassion or *agape*

My remit is to study the relevance of truth-telling in relation to trust, but the relevance of compassion or empathy merits a brief mention. Several authors articulate the need for compassion or empathy in order for trust to develop in the doctor–patient relationship.[38] Smith and Churchill provide us with a good definition of compassion.

> Compassion is not saccharine pity or demeaning self-righteousness to the less fortunate; neither is it associated with the charisma which forms part of the physician's traditional authority. [...] Authentic compassion, on the other hand, engages one genuinely and empathetically in community with another.[39]

Competence is an important attribute for inspiring confidence, but compassion offers the hope that those other dimensions of illness – emotional and spiritual – will also be attended to. Carl Rudebeck, a Swedish GP, describes empathy as 'the ability to grasp the lived experience of the body – the existential anatomy – of another person'.[40] Illness is almost always a threat, a crisis, particularly when the outcome is uncertain. To reach out to a steady hand extended to one when crossing the turbulent waters can give solace, solidarity and hope.

In the film *The Doctor*, John Hurt plays a prima donna thoracic consultant who succumbs to throat cancer. His (female) surgeon is competent and frank (brutally so), yet utterly devoid of warmth or empathy. In the end, he switches to the 'soft' humanistic surgeon, whom he knows is both compassionate and competent – a man who would be willing to 'go the extra mile', and not abandon him to a miserable, lonely fate. In short, a man he can trust to *care* (even though the hero had ridiculed him earlier in his healthy days).

The doctor–patient relationship: models

The doctor–patient relationship forms the bedrock of general practice. It is seen as having both instrumental and intrinsic value[41, 42] and is connected to a holistic, person-centred view rather than a biomedical, disease-centred perspective.[43] Rogers and Braunack-Mayer give practical as well as moral reasons why trust is of value in the doctor–patient relationship suggesting that communication is easier (less need to check up on or challenge what is said), with less anxiety about what can be said (and anyone faced with a hostile sceptical patient can testify to this), and the goals of the consultation can be more readily defined. The GP can have more discretionary latitude and there is more scope for tolerating uncertainty as well as greater flexibility to meet the changing demands brought on by the patient's variable needs. They stress the need for mutual trust and emphasise the need for doctors to be prepared to trust and fully listen, to bear witness to the patient's testimony. Whilst acknowledging that there is a risk of misplacing that trust from time to time, they conclude:

> Trust plays a crucial role, both moral and practical, in doctor–patient relationships. [...] There is an obligation for the GPs to consciously, and demonstrably, be trustworthy, and to trust patients unless there are justifiable reasons for not trusting.[44]

If we conclude that trust is the cornerstone of relationships, which of the many different models for the doctor–patient relationship is the most strongly linked to trust? There is an overwhelming multiplicity of models. By placing them under the umbrella of different meta-ethical systems, this diversity becomes more manageable.

The engineering, business, contractual or consumerist model

In this model, the doctor provides a service to the client–consumer, who is presumed to be autonomous and well-informed, and knows what he or she wants. The doctor delivers the service competently, effectively abdicating responsibility for decisions, apart from technical ones as to how to achieve the desired result (of the patient). An example of this might be a surgeon practising private plastic surgery for wealthy healthy clients, or surgeons and doctors working in 'boutique medicine'. In this model, healthcare is viewed as a commodity to be bought by users and sold by providers. In spirit, it is competitive rather than collaborative. There is little scope for true dialogue or shared agreement. Respect for autonomy is narrowly defined by ensuring that the criteria for informed consent are fulfilled. This is a dangerous position, as it suggests that the profession has no normative goals.[45] Consumerism is closely linked to the advent of a rights-based philosophy in modern Western society (discussed in greater detail in Chapter 4). There is considerable discussion as to where rights originate and various theories have been put forward.[46] I shall not be discussing these here. Suffice to say that rights are worthless – like actors strutting on an empty stage – unless there is an agent that has both the obligation and the capacity to fulfil those rights. A right to healthcare, for example, is of little use in a country where there are insufficient resources to provide even basic healthcare needs.

Libertarian philosophies, with their emphasis on individual autonomy, do not incorporate trusting relationships in their frameworks. The individual who is totally independent-minded, possessing individual autonomy in high measure, may inspire admiration, but not trust. Will he be there for you if helping you jeopardises his self-interests? The *chacun pour soi* mentality does not allow for connectedness or for duties to one another.

> Trust flourishes between those who are linked to one another; individual autonomy flourishes where everyone has 'space' to do their own thing. Trust belongs with relationships and (mutual) obligations; individual autonomy with rights and adversarial claims.[47]

The consumerist model is truly incoherent for it allows for one individual – the health professional – to be used 'merely as a means', but not as 'an end', to paraphrase Kant's moral imperative. If both parties share the same end, there is no real difficulty. The problem arises if there is a divergence. With the consumerist model, there is no dialogue or meaningful conversation – no thrashing out of a consensus. The patient engages with the doctor, not as a person, but as an instrument – and yet, paradoxically, the assumption (or trust!) is that the doctor will not reciprocate by treating the patient instrumentally. The doctor's professional role is deemed to eclipse his or her individual autonomy. But how can one guarantee this? This uncertainty fosters the consumer–patient's mistrust. And what impact will this type of encounter have on the doctor? The betting is that he or she will be left feeling angry, 'used' and mistrustful. This, I believe, is the fundamental problem with 'positive' rights, rather than the 'negative' rights (the right to non-interference) described by John Stuart Mill:[48] it forces others to fulfil your wishes, even if doing so contravenes their own autonomous wishes and values. Kant's categorical imperative is consensual in that it enjoins the rational person to act only on maxims, which he would will to have universalised.[49] Clearly we would not want others to coerce us to act on their behalf in ways that we deem to be unethical. The other major problem with this model is that it assumes all patients are rational and autonomous 'consumers', and ignores the vulnerability and dependency of those whose autonomy is impaired by physical or mental illness, fear or senility, or of those, such as children, who have not developed autonomy. Arguably these groups form a large proportion of doctors' clientele and are precisely the groups whose trust is particularly vulnerable to abuse.

> But equality is not even a desirable ideal in all relationships [...] and we need a morality to guide us in our dealings with those who cannot or should not achieve equality of power (animals, the ill, the dying, children whilst still young) with those with whom they have unavoidable and often intimate relationships.[50]

The contractual model

This model, favoured by Veatch,[51] is essentially a variant of the consumerist model and views both doctor and patient as equal partners in a commodity transaction. Rights and duties are expressed within a legalistic framework in which trust plays a minimal role. This model has been robustly critiqued by Christie and Hoffmaster,[52] Annette Baier[53] and Howard Brody.[54] The problems have been identified as:

- doctors and patients rarely begin relationships on contractual terms
- the framework is too rigid and legalistic to allow for varying clinical needs
- the importance of the integrity of the ongoing relationship as it evolves is denied
- the fact of illness may impair autonomy and creates vulnerability
- the focus on patient autonomy is too narrow

- the doctor–patient dyad is viewed in isolation rather than embedded in social systems
- minimalist 'bottom-line' thinking is encouraged, rather than fostering relationships that enhance patient welfare.

This model is therefore also based on mistrust, not trust. Baier, in her perceptive essay, points out how the great moral theorists neglected trust and explains this as a reflection of a 'male fixation on contract' and an impoverished abstract view of relationships: 'Modern moral philosophy has concentrated on the morality of fairly cool relationships between those who are deemed to be roughly equal in power to determine the rules and to instigate sanctions against rule breakers.'[55]

The apostolic, paternalistic, 'doctor-centred' model

In this model the doctor is the 'wise expert' and the patient abdicates responsibility, allowing the doctor to dictate the management that he or she believes will best serve the patient. This is a reversal of the consumerist model. The emphasis is on beneficence (as decided by the doctor) rather than patient autonomy. The patient is not encouraged or allowed to enact his or her autonomy. There is no real mutuality or engagement with the patient's values, beliefs or preferences. Strong paternalism may occasionally be necessary if the patient is too ill to exert his or her autonomy and the patient's beliefs and preferences are not known. In this acute situation, the doctor is expected to use his or her knowledge or skills, and practical wisdom. This is an example of Szasz and Hollander's 'activity-passivity' model.[56]

The public health model

This is an extension of the apostolic model, adopting a consequentialist framework that goes beyond the individual. Central to the model is the objective of maximising health, measured by epidemiological markers such as mortality or morbidity rates. It is underpinned by a mechanistic view of human health and aims for the 'greatest good for the greatest number', eschewing concerns for individual autonomy. The imposition of health targets in primary care has led to an inevitable clash with the individualist–consumerist viewpoint, as well as to public mistrust, particularly when such targets were found to be linked to financial incentives for GPs. The disease, not the patient, is the focus and individuals are used instrumentally for the benefit of the 'common good'. Peter Toon argues that 'This model gives scope for an almost infinite medicalisation of life' with corresponding limitless responsibilities for doctors and that 'there is a tendency for paternalism and even authoritarianism'.[57]

'Mutuality' models

Pellegrino and Thomasma argue for a model where health functions as a relational good – a prominent value for both patient and doctor, acting as moral agents in relation to one another. They coin the term 'beneficence-in-trust' as respecting patient autonomy whilst making a benefits-to-burdens calculation about the quality of a person's life. They link the 'act of the profession' with 'the fact of illness'; the latter viewed as an ontological assault, threatening the integrity of the sick person.[58] They argue that their framework is not fully represented by utilitarian or deontological principles, and later attempt to combine their model with Virtue Theory[59] (*see* below). They do this unsuccessfully, in my view, as the virtues are 'added-on' in an arbitrary way, rather than being integral as in Aristotle's meta-ethical theory.[60] Arguably their model is primarily deontological, founded on the Kantian maxim 'to treat persons as ends in themselves, rather than merely as a means', with an enriched perspective on the phenomenological experience of illness.

Zaner endorses 'togetherness and mutuality' rather than 'insularity and autonomy' as defining our existence, and implicitly critiques Kant. For Zaner, the doctor–patient relationship is based on trust:

> trust in the context of initial, vital vulnerability and diminish-ment of selfhood [...] The therapeutic dyad of trust and care has its basis, on the one hand in the 'moral chance' of illness and in the scientifically and linguistically informed clinical act of affil-iative feeling, on the other.[61]

Other models of the relationship, such as Balint's hermeneutic model,[62] Buber's I and thou relationship,[63] Bauman's post-modern ethics,[64] Emanuel and Emanuel's deliberative relationship,[65] Szasz and Hollender's mutual participatory model,[66] not to mention the patient-centred method of Stewart and McWhinney,[67] all stress reciprocity, and, to a greater or lesser extent, the virtues.

The covenantal model is likewise based on reciprocity. A covenant is defined by McWhinney as 'an undertaking to do whatever is needed, even if it means going beyond the contract'.[68] This model, grounded in the religious notion of man's covenant with God, is open-ended, unlike a con-tract, and freely engaged upon. It was developed by May[69] in the context of medicine and has been widely adopted by others. Campbell describes the covenantal relationship as promoting trust and mutuality, and requiring 'bodily mediation in order for its true value to be appropriated by helped and helper alike'.[70] Even Onora O'Neill's Kantian concept of 'principled autonomy' emphasises mutuality.

In all these models, trust looms large – indeed, is intrinsic to them. They reflect the essence of those more intimate relationships and friendships we have in other parts of our lives.

A virtue/narrative-based model of the doctor–patient relationship

In his important book, *After Virtue,* Alasdair MacIntyre modernised and revitalised Aristotle's virtue ethics, and stressed the criticality of narrative. The individual is viewed as author of his or her life. Rather than asking the question 'What ought I to do?' we ask 'What kind of person do I wish to be? What story or stories am I part of?' Personal identity is founded on 'an integrated life-narrative which we tell ourselves and which we present to the world as part of a larger shared tradition'.[71] He defines the virtues in this way:

> The virtues therefore are to be understood as those dispositions which will not only sustain practices and enable us to achieve the good internal to practices, but which will also sustain us in the relevant kind of quest for the good, by enabling us to overcome the harms, dangers, temptations and distractions which we encounter, and which will furnish us with increasing self-knowledge and increasing knowledge of the good.[72]

The virtuous physician, in this schema, will be honest and possess integrity. Virtue ethics, it should be added, is not a recipe for burnout, as balance, or temperance is also a key virtue. Peter Toon gives a clear and detailed discussion of the virtuous practitioner, and I shall not dwell further on the topic.[73]

Narrative ethics insists that we attend to the richness and complexity of experience. Arthur Frank says: 'Thinking *with* stories is the basis of narrative ethics. Stories are the ongoing work of turning mere existence into a life that is social, and moral, and affirms the existence of the teller as a human being'.[74]

Patients are often vulnerable and may, in reality, have few choices. They have to cope with uncertainty, amongst other burdens, and without a clear outcome. They suffer from a loss of trust in their bodies and their wellbeing. Their social roles are threatened. Suddenly and catastrophically, the road ahead becomes blurred, chaotic and even meaningless. Frank describes this threat of disintegration and loss of purpose as 'narrative wreckage'. He describes three broad pathways for illness narratives: chaos, restitution and quest. Restitution is the reclamation or restoration of the self and quest refers to illness becoming transformational – a catalyst for change – enriching, rather than impoverishing, the sufferer's life. Howard Brody likens illness to a 'broken story'.[75] For both Frank and Brody, the doctor's role is to help the patient create a new and meaningful story. For Frank, the patient has the moral responsibility to give testimony of his suffering to the community and the doctor has the duty to bear witness to it. Empathy involves the recognition that we are all vulnerable and incomplete.

What reinforces or erodes trust? The empirical evidence

Do narrative ethics encompass and foster trust? Proponents would vigorously affirm that they do. Certainly the evidence suggests that listening to the patient's story and working with it appears to promote trust. One of the problems is finding a valid and reliable instrument to measure trust. Some researchers have attempted to do so. Their studies suggest that patients' trust in their doctors is strongly associated with the quality of the GP–patient relationship, including communication, interpersonal care and knowledge of the patient.[76]

Trust also appears to matter in terms of outcomes: patients with low trust were less satisfied with the care provided, were less likely to adhere to the advice given and had less symptom improvement.[77, 78] Little is known about the process whereby trust is developed in the relationship.[79] There is conflicting evidence that one of the crucial factors for trust is continuity of care and personal knowledge of the physician.[80] More important appears to be the quality of the relationship with the GP, rather than the number of times the patient has seen the GP. This relationship will become more difficult with the evolution of large practices, part-time practitioners and the emphasis on immediate access. The evidence suggests that managed care in the USA and the (now extinct) variant in the UK – individual Fundholding – damages trust.[81, 82]

Conclusion

So where does this leave us? Allowing for some fuzziness at the boundaries of the different models of the doctor–patient relationship, we can state with confidence that the consumerist ethic, with the primacy of individual autonomy, and the concurrent paternalistic utilitarian ethic are running a collision course. Furthermore, both models are inimical to trust. The other models founded on reciprocity, narrative and virtue hold greater promise for trust and the doctor–patient relationship. Perhaps we should abandon attempts to adhere rigidly to one model, as suggested by Greg Clarke.[83] But Clarke's critique is based on a narrow area of decision-making with regard to treatment and a narrow concept of what philosophies the models represent. Furthermore, it is clear that rarely will the consumerist model or the paternalistic model of care be applicable in the context of general practice. Broadly, the moral life of GPs in their practices more closely resembles that of lay people in their everyday lives: a broad tapestry woven with subtle challenges and perplexities, frequent interactions as well as long-term relationships – these bringing with them their own particular responsibilities and constraints. GPs endeavour to share their medical expertise with patients' personal knowledge and experience of their illnesses in an ongoing dialogue.[84, 85]

Truthfulness and truth-telling

Truth-telling as harmful

> Truth is the breath of life to human society. It is the food of the immortal spirit. Yet a single word of it may kill a man as suddenly as a drop of prussic acid.[86]

Confidentiality and truth-telling are two sides of the same coin – they represent the power to control information.[87] Yet the emphasis for many centuries has been on confidentiality, not truth-telling – indeed, truth-telling has been proscribed and viewed as harmful to the patient. For example, the Hippocratic oath urges physicians to preserve confidences, but advises against telling the truth for fear of damaging patients' health. Until quite recently, truthfulness has not featured in medical or nursing professional codes of conduct. The importance of telling the truth to patients is a relatively recent phenomenon. In her book, *Lying*,[88] Sissela Bok attributes this change to the emergence of the concept of informed consent, as does Sheila McLean.[89]

With the demise of traditional paternalism, it is dubious whether doctors can justify lying to patients with the aim of protecting them from harm. As Roger Higgs argues, 'harm is a very personal concept' and should not be decided by the doctor.[90] He argues that we should distinguish between the abstract concept of truth (of which we may always have an incomplete grasp) and *telling* the truth as we know it 'where the *intention* is all important'. He questions the justifications for not telling patients the truth, notably the principles of beneficence and non-maleficence, and says doctors can hide behind these to disguise their own discomfort, avoiding truthful disclosure to protect themselves from confronting death and painful emotions. He argues that deceit is detrimental to the patient's health and concludes that telling the truth is essential to the health of the doctor–patient relationship. Doctors should not assume that patients cannot cope with a diagnosis of a life-threatening illness – the elderly, in particular, may be more philosophical in this context.

But *how* we tell the truth forms part of the moral dimension. 'Centuries of systematic insensitive deception cannot be remedied by a new routine of systematic insensitive truth-telling' argues the oncologist, Robert Buckman.[91] Breaking bad news is an important, necessary and always challenging part of medical work, requiring skill and sensitivity.

Truthfulness as a virtue

> This above all – to Thine own sense be true,
> And it must follow, as the night the day,
> Thou canst not then be false to any man.[92]

> Polonius to Laertes, *Hamlet*, Act I, scene 3

Bernard Williams, in detailed analysis of truthfulness, identifies two virtues: accuracy and sincerity. Accuracy is the virtue of carefully investigating and deliberating over the evidence before accepting it as truth and sincerity is the virtue of genuinely expressing to others what one believes to be the truth. Williams argues that accurate and sincere communication between persons is necessary for the development of trust and facilitates human flourishing.[93]

The empirical evidence

But what do patients actually want? In the 1980s, empirical studies showed that over 90% of patients wished to be informed if they had cancer.[94] In 1996, Meredith *et al* showed that nearly 80% wished to know as much as possible about their condition and 96% if their illness was cancer.[95] In addition, Benson and Britten's study showed that nearly two-thirds of patients felt, with a few exceptions, that family members should not be told the diagnosis without explicit consent.[96] Nevertheless there was a small, but significant minority who did *not* wish to be informed.

There may also be cultural differences to truth-telling, and we should take note of anecdotal stories describing how 'giving up hope' may have contributed to an early demise. For example, Hassan and Hassan describe how seven patients with cancer died unexpectedly within 48 hours of being told there was 'no hope of cure'.[97]

Distinguishing between lying, deceiving and concealing

> The first rule is to speak the truth; the second is to speak with discretion.

Blaise Pascal

In her substantive and cogently argued book, *Truth, Trust and Medicine*, Jennifer Jackson submits that with the current medical teaching, the distinct acts of lying, deceiving and concealing tend to be conflated, such that the duty not to lie becomes a *prima facie* duty to be weighed against (and readily overridden by) others. Similarly, truthfulness is conflated with frankness and openness. And, as she argues, 'it is so obviously impossible, and anyway improper, to be frank and open always', thus both frankness *and* truthfulness become discretionary. She argues for a narrow but strict definition of lying such that the teaching should repudiate lying altogether. Truthfulness is needed to sustain trust and respect. This teaching 'Is the only teaching that is adequate to sustain trust [...] That trust is and always has been a necessary supporting pillar of the covenant between the patient and health professional. That is the essence of truthfulness as a virtue.'[98]

As with other virtues, this is something that we constantly aspire to and hone with practice. But we should also be cautious in what we disclose – this skill requires practical wisdom, or judgment – Aristotle's *phronesis* – gained from reflecting on experience.[99] O'Neill takes the same view, but expresses it differently: she argues that to increase trust we need to avoid deception rather than secrecy. She questions whether transparency can protect us from deceit.

> Increasing transparency can produce a flood of unsorted information and misinformation that provides little but confusion unless it can be sorted and assessed. It may add to uncertainty rather than to trust [...] Transparency can encourage people to be less honest, so increasing deception and reducing reasons for trust: those who know *everything* they say or write is to be made public may massage the truth [...] Demands for universal transparency are likely to encourage the evasions, hypocrisies and half-truths that we usually refer to as 'political correctness', but which might more forthrightly be called either 'self-censorship' or 'deception'.[100]

Jennifer Jackson concludes that lying is always wrong, except in extreme circumstances where life or limb are at stake and that lying must be distinguished from concealment, and truth-telling from candour. I agree with her that if we use these distinctions, we gain greater moral clarity and rigour in our communications. But at what stage should doctors share their concerns? Arguably, a 'hunch' or suspicion is materially different from a firm diagnosis.

> A doctor awaiting test results does not yet have information. This is not an instance of defensible deception because there is no deceiving, no attempt to make the patient believe what is false; only intent to conceal. It is an instance of (defensible) concealment. The concealment might be indefensible – if, say, it is obviously causing the patient undue anxiety – but it is not a failure of truthfulness.[101]

Howard Brody, however, is more implacable and views withholding information just as culpable as deception: 'Withholding that information, because it short-circuits any possibility of meaningful free choice, is a very special way of displaying a basic disrespect for moral dignity and personhood of someone else.'[102]

I tend to agree with Jackson that doctors may be acting ethically if they conceal hunches and expectations until the results of tests confirm them – otherwise they may be needlessly (or cruelly) fuelling fears. But on the other hand, exploring hidden fears should be part of the dialogue (otherwise they will fester, undisclosed): if a patient expresses fear of cancer or any other worrying diagnosis, the GP then has the opportunity to reassure the patient that these are unlikely, but should be ruled out. Indeed, it would be negligent not to do so.

Deception regarding *certain* information is another matter. By deceiving 'we make others our victims, and undermine or distort their possibilities for acting and communicating.'[103] In *The Death of Ivan Ilyich*, Tolstoy eloquently describes the betrayal, isolation and anguish of a man who knows he is dying, but whose family and doctors persist in maintaining the deception that he is not.

> And the pretence made him wretched: it tormented him that they refused to admit what they knew and he knew to be a fact, but persisted in lying to him concerning his terrible condition, and wanted him and forced him to be party to the lie. Deceit, this deceit enacted over him up to the very eve of his death: this lying which could only degrade the awful solemn act of his death to the level of their visitings, their curtains, their sturgeon for dinner [...] was horribly painful to Ivan Ilyich.[104]

Conclusion

Trust is ineradicable in human relationships. Truthfulness is a necessary, albeit insufficient, ingredient of trust. GPs should strive to be accurate and sincere if they truly respect their patients and value their own authenticity. They need, however, to distinguish carefully candour and openness from lying and intentional deception.

The doctor–patient relationship that is most conducive to trust is one of mutual engagement and respect. The relationship most inimical to trust is the one whereby individuals are treated instrumentally. This 'ethics of distrust' is flawed empirically, phenomenologically and conceptually. The consumerist individualistic model is ultimately self-defeating and the utilitarian preventative model unsustainable.

GPs hunker down in the privacy of their consulting rooms to maintain good, patient-centred general practice. 'And it is precisely here, in the consultation, that the GP has an exceptional potential for trust: in the capacity of personal doctoring.'[105] But for how long can they keep threatening forces out of the consulting room? For the consumerist model is becoming more powerful and more pervasive. The public (fuelled by the media and government agendas) are becoming more vocal in their perceived entitlements. 'Patient choice', not 'patient need', is the dominant slogan. Empowerment, not vulnerability, is emphasised. Individuality displaces solidarity. I have not even addressed other current threats in my discussion, such as the erosion of confidentiality and the fragmentation of care.

Whether we like it or not, we are undergoing a paradigm shift. The challenge is to maintain the core values of good general practice that are cherished by both the professionals and the lay public. It seems to me to be essential to grasp what paradigm we are shifting into so that we can be critically aware of its moral and professional implications. Gauging the current socio-political scene, I think it is reasonable to surmise that general practice and trust are in crisis. If we really care about our patients, we should join forces and creatively resist unbridled consumerism and utilitarian medicine. Any philosophical model for the doctor–patient relationship needs to reflect the goals of medicine and the lived experience of general practice. In the end, trust, not rights, will trump.

References

1 Brazier M, Lobjoit M. Fiduciary relationship: an ethical approach and legal concept? In: Bennett R and Erin CA, editors. *HIV and AIDS Testing, Screening and Confidentiality*. Oxford: Oxford University Press; 1999.

2 O' Hara K. *Trust. From Socrates to Spin*. Cambridge: Icon Books; 2004. p. 14.

3 Fugelli P. Trust – in general practice. *BJGP*. 2001; **51**: 575–9.

4 Williams B. *Truth and Truthfulness. An essay in genealogy*. Princeton: Princeton University Press; 2004.

5 Blackburn S. *Truth. A guide for the perplexed*. London: Allan Lane; 2005.

6 O'Hara K. *Ibid*. p. 9.

7 Etchells R. Listening to literature. In: Harrison J, Innes R, van Zwanenberg T, eds. *Rebuilding Trust in Healthcare*. Oxford: Radcliffe Medical Press; 2003.

8 Baier A. Trust and antitrust. In: *Moral Prejudices. Essays on ethics*. Cambridge, MA and London: Harvard University Press; 1994. p. 95.

9 Fugelli P. Trust – in general practice. *BJGP*. 2001; **51**: 575–9.

10 Luhmann N. *Trust and Power*. New York: John Wiley; 1979.

11 Luhmann N. *Ibid*. p. 39.

12 Seligman AB. *The Problem of Trust*. Princeton: Princeton University Press; 1997. p. 21.

13 http://www.the-hutton-inquiry.org.uk/content/report/

14 O'Neill O. *A Question of Trust. The BBC Reith Lectures*. Cambridge: Cambridge University Press; 2002. p. 57.

15 Emmet D. *Rules, Roles and Relations*. London: St Martin's Press; 1967.

16 Emmet D. *Ibid*. p. 183.

17 Seligman AB. *The Problem of Trust*. Princeton: Princeton University Press; 1997.

18 Taylor D, Leese B. Recruitment, retention, and time commitment change in general practitioners in England and Wales 1990–4: a retrospective survey. *BMJ*. 1997; **314**: 1806–10.

19 *The Declaration of Geneva*, adopted by the World Medical Association, 1948. www.wma.net/e/policy/c8.htm

20 Lifton RJ. *The Nazi Doctors: medical killing and the psychology of genocide*. New York: Basic Books; 1986.

21 Lifton RJ. Doctors and torture. *NEJM*. 2004; **351**: 415–6.

22 MORI poll, 2004. Mori.com/polls/2004/bma.shtml

23 O'Neill O. *A Question of Trust. The BBC Reith Lectures*. Cambridge: Cambridge University Press; 2002. p. 19.

24 Harvey D. *Condition of Postmodernity*. Cambridge: Basil Blackwell; 1989.

25 Seligman AB. *The Problem of Trust*. Princeton: Princeton University Press; 1997. p. 154.

26 Seligman AB. *Ibid*. p. 165.

27 Seligman AB. *Ibid*. p. 174.

28 Bauman Z. *Liquid Love. On the frailty of human bonds*. Cambridge: Polity Press; 2003. p. 88–9.

29 MacIntyre A. *After Virtue. A study in moral theory*. 2nd ed. London: Duckworth; 1985. p. 55.

30 MacIntyre A. *Ibid*. p. 55.

31 For example: *The Patient in the Family. The ethics of medicine and families*. Lindemann Nelson HL and Lindemann Nelson J. London: Routledge; 1995. Parker M. *Ethics and Community in the Healthcare Professions*. London: Routledge; 1999.

32 For example: Brody H. *Stories of Sickness*. London: Yale University Press: 1987. Frank AW. *The Wounded Storyteller. Body, illness and ethics*. Chicago: University

of Chicago Press; 1995. Lindemann Nelson HL, editor. *Stories and Their Limits. Narrative approaches to bioethics.* London: Routledge; 1997. Charon R, Montello M, editors. *Stories Matter. The role of narrative in medical ethics.* London: Routledge; 2002.

33 Horton R. *Second Opinion. Doctors, diseases and decisions in modern medicine.* London: Granta Books; 2003. p. 40.

34 Horton R. *Ibid.* p. r43.

35 Diamond J. *C: Because cowards get cancer too.* London: Vermillion; 1998. p. 40.

36 Editorial. Helping the informed patient decide. *The Lancet.* 2005; **365**: 2064.

37 Editorial. Herceptin and early breast cancer: a moment for caution. *The Lancet.* 2005; **366**: 1673.

38 For example: Halpern J. *From Detached Concern to Empathy. Humanizing medical practice.* Oxford: Oxford University Press; 2001. Spiro R, editor. *Empathy and the Practice of Medicine.* New Haven: Yale University Press; 1993.

39 Smith HL, Churchill LR. *Professional Ethics and Primary Care Medicine. Beyond dilemmas and decorum.* Durham: Duke University Press; 1986. p. 50.

40 Rudebeck CE. Imagination and empathy in the consultation. *BJGP.* 2002; **52**: 450–3.

41 McWhinney IR. *A Textbook of Family Medicine.* 2nd ed. Oxford: Oxford University Press; 1997.

42 Christie RJ, Hoffmaster CB. *Ethical Issues in Family Medicine.* Oxford: Oxford University Press; 1986.

43 Toon P. *What is Good General Practice?* London: Royal College of General Practitioners, Occasional Paper 65; 1994. p. 34.

44 Rogers W, Braunack-Mayer A. *A Practical Ethics for General Practice.* Oxford: Oxford University Press; 2004. p. 25.

45 Gormally L, editor. *Issues for a Catholic Bioethic.* London: Linacre Centre; 1999.

46 For example, Dworkin R. *Taking Rights Seriously.* London: Duckworths; 1996. Waldron J, editor. *Theories of Rights.* Oxford: Oxford University Press; 1984.

47 O'Neill O. *A Question of Trust. The BBC Reith Lectures.* Cambridge: Cambridge University Press; 2002. p. 25

48 Mill JS. *On Liberty.* In: *'On Liberty' and Other Writings* (Cambridge Texts in the History of Political Thought). Cambridge: Cambridge University Press; 1989.

49 Kant I. *Groundwork of the Metaphysics of Morals.* (Trans. by Paton HJ). London: Harper and Row; 1964.

50 Baier AC. Trust and antitrust. In: *Moral Prejudices. Essays on ethics.* Cambridge, MA and London: Harvard University Press; 1994. p. 116.

51 Veatch R. *A Theory of Medical Ethics.* New York: Basic Books; 1981.

52 Christie RJ, Hoffmaster CB. *Ethical Issues in Family Medicine.* Oxford: Oxford University Press; 1986.

53 Baier AC. Trust and antitrust. In: *Moral Prejudices. Essays on ethics.* Cambridge, MA and London: Harvard University Press; 1994.

54 Brody H. The physician/patient relationship. In: Veatch RM, editor. *Medical Ethics.* Boston: Jones and Bartlett; 1989.

55 Baier AC. Trust and antitrust. In: *Moral Prejudices. Essays on ethics.* Cambridge, MA and London: Harvard University Press; 1994. p. 116.

56 Szasz TS and Hollander MH. The basic models of the doctor–patient relationship. *AMA Archives of Internal Medicine.* 1956; **97**: 585.

57 Toon P. *What is Good General Practice?* London: Royal College of General Practioners, Occasional Paper 65; 1994. p. 34.

58 Pellegrino ED, Thomasma DC. *For the Patient's Good. The restoration of beneficence in healthcare.* Oxford: Oxford University Press; 1988.

59 Pellegrino ED, Thomasma DC. *The Virtues in Medical Practice.* Oxford: Oxford University Press; 1993.

60 Aristotle. In: Thomson JAK, translator. *Nichomachean Ethics.* London: Penguin Books; 1953.

61 Zaner RM. *Ethics and the Clinical Encounter.* New Jersey: Prentice Hall; 1988.

62 Balint M. *The Doctor, his Patient and the Illness.* London: Pitman Medical; 1964.

63 Buber M. *I and Thou.* 2nd ed. London: Continuum; 1958.

64 Bauman Z. *Postmodern Ethics.* Oxford: Blackwell; 1993.

65 Emanuel EJ, Emanuel LL. Four models of the physician–patient relationship. *JAMA.* 1992; **267**: 2221–6.

66 Szasz TS, Hollender MH. The basic models of the doctor–patient relationship. *AMA Archives of Internal Medicine.* 1956; **97**: 585.

67 Stewart M *et al. Patient-Centered Medicine. Transforming the clinical method.* 2nd ed. Oxford: Radcliffe Medical Press; 2003.

68 McWhinney I. Core values in a changing world. *BMJ.* 1998; **316**: 1807–9.

69 May WF. *The Physician's Covenant – images of the healer in medical ethics.* Philadelphia: Westminster Press; 1983.

70 Campbell AV. *Moderated Love. A theology of professional care.* London: SPCK Publishing; 1984.

71 MacIntyre A. *After Virtue. A study in moral theory.* 2nd ed. London: Duckworth; 1985. p. 221.

72 MacIntyre A. *Ibid.* p. 219.

73 Toon PD. *Towards a Philosophy of General Practice: a study of the virtuous practitioner.* London: Royal College of General Practitioners, Occasional Paper 78; 1999.

74 Frank A. *The Wounded Storyteller. Body, illness and ethics.* London: University of Chicago Press; 1995.

75 Brody H. *Stories of Sickness.* London: Yale University Press; 1987.

76 Tarrant C, Stokes T, Baker R. Factors associated with patients' trust in their general practitioner: a cross-sectional survey. *BJGP.* 2003; **53**: 798–800.

77 Thom DH *et al.* Patient trust in the physician: relationship to patient requests. *Family Practice.* 2002; **19**: 476–83.

78 Safran DG, Taira DA, Rogers WH. Linking primary care performances to outcomes of care. *J Fam Pract.* 1998; **47**: 213–20.

79 Pearson SD, Raeke LH. Patients' trust in physicians: many theories, few measures, little data. *J Gen Intern Med.* 2000; **15**: 509–13.

80 Mainous AG III, Baker R, Love MM *et al.* Continuity of care and trust in one's physician: evidence from primary care in the United States and the United Kingdom. *Fam Med.* 2001; **33**: 22–7.

81 Simon SR *et al.* Views of managed care – a survey of students, residents, faculty and deans at medical schools in the United States. *NEJM.* **340**: 928–36.

82 Smith LFP, Morrissey JR. Ethical dilemmas for general practitioners under the new UK contract. *JME*. 1994; **20**: 175–80.

83 Clarke G. Physician-patient relations: no more models. *AJOB*. 2004; **4**(2): 16–19.

84 Stewart M, Brown JB, Weston WW *et al*. *Patient-Centered Medicine. Transforming the clinical method*. 2nd ed. Oxford: Radcliffe Medical Press; 2003.

85 Rogers W. Beneficence in general practice – empirical observation. *JME*. 1999; **25**: 388–93.

86 Holmes OW. Valedictory Address 1858, Harvard Commencement.

87 Brody H. *The Healer's Power*. New Haven: Yale University Press; 1992.

88 Bok S. *Lying*. Hassocks: The Harvester Press; 1978.

89 McLean S. *A Patient's Right to Know*. Aldershot: Dartmouth; 1989.

90 Higgs R. On telling patients the truth. In: Lockwood M, editor. *Moral Dilemmas in Medicine*. Oxford: Oxford University Press; 1988.

91 Buckman R. Talking to patients about cancer. *BMJ*. 1996; **313**: 699–700.

92 Shakespeare W. *Hamlet*, Act 1, scene 3.

93 Williams B. *Truth and Truthfulness. An essay in genealogy*. Princeton: Princeton University Press; 2004.

94 Northouse P, Northouse LLO. Communication and cancer issues confronting patients, health professionals and family members. *J Psychosocial Oncol*. 1987; **5**: 17–45.

95 Meredith C, Symonds P, Webster L *et al*. Information needs of cancer patients in the west of Scotland. *BMJ*. 1996; **313**: 724–6.

96 Benson J, Britten N. How much truth and to whom? Respecting the autonomy of cancer patients when talking to their families – ethical theory and the patients' view. *BMJ*. 1996; **313**: 729–31.

97 Hassan AMF, Hassan A. Do we always need to tell patients the truth? *The Lancet*. 1998; **352**: 1153.

98 Jackson J. *Truth, Trust and Medicine*. London: Routledge; 2001. p. 157.

99 Aristotle. In: Thomson JAK, translator; revised by Treddenick H. *Nichomachean Ethics*. London: Penguin Classics; 1976. For a modern and readable account of virtue ethics, *see also* Hursthouse R. *On Virtue Ethics*. Oxford: Oxford University Press; 1999.

100 O'Neill O. *A Question of Trust. The BBC Reith Lectures*. Cambridge: Cambridge University Press; 2002. p. 72–3.

101 Jackson J. *Truth, Trust and Medicine*. London: Routledge; 2001.

102 Brody H. *The Physician/Patient Relationship*. In: *Medical Ethics*: Veatch RM, editor. Boston: Jones and Bartlett; 1989. p. 80.

103 O'Neill O. *A Question of Trust: The BBC Reith Lectures*. Cambridge: Cambridge University Press; 2002. p. 96–7.

104 Tolstoy L. *The Death of Ivan Ilyich*. London: Penguin Books; 1960/95.

105 Fugelli P. Trust – in general practice. *BJGP*. 2001; **51**: 177.

Chapter 2

Autonomy and paternalism in primary care

Margaret Lloyd

> No Man is an Island.
>
> John Donne

Introduction

Respect for autonomy has become the major guiding principle in healthcare ethics. This may not always be in the interest of the patient and society, and many consider that the balance between autonomy and paternalism has swung too much in favour of autonomy. In this chapter, these issues will be addressed by examining some of the theoretical concepts of autonomy and paternalism, and applying them to situations that arise in primary care. Issues of confidentiality and truth-telling are relevant to a consideration of autonomy and paternalism, but the main emphasis will be on decision-making within the consultation.

To begin with, consider the issues raised by the following case studies. Think about what 'autonomy' and 'respect for autonomy' mean for you and then think about which of the patients has autonomy, how their autonomy can be respected and when paternalistic care is appropriate.

Case studies

Ms A, a 35-year-old woman with Down's syndrome, has severe menorrhagia which has not been controlled by medical treatment. The gynaecologist has recommended that she has a hysterectomy. Ms A and her mother come to discuss this with you. She does not want to have the operation but her mother thinks that it's a 'good idea'.

Mr B is a 56-year-old advertising executive with diabetes and high serum cholesterol who continues to smoke 25 cigarettes a day. During a visit to the diabetic clinic, he says that he has not been taking his simvastatin and, although he would like to stop smoking, he has decided that he enjoys it too much to stop.

Ms C is aged 40 and pregnant for the fifth time, having had two abortions and complications in one of her previous deliveries. She is insisting that she has a right to have a home birth and has asked to see her practice records.

Mrs D has insulin-dependent diabetes. Whilst waiting for her appointment at the diabetic clinic she collapses after complaining to the receptionist of feeling cold and dizzy. The GP diagnoses hypoglycaemia and gives her intravenous glucose and intramuscular glucagon.

Mrs E has breast cancer and has had surgery and radiotherapy. The oncologist has strongly recommended chemotherapy rather than tamoxifen. Mrs E tells her GP that she doesn't want to be involved in this decision and wants to leave it to the doctors caring for her. Moreover she doesn't want to know the results of any further tests.

Mrs G, a former teacher in her early fifties, has motor neurone disease and is terminally ill with respiratory failure. Her GP has looked after her for many years and is disturbed when she refuses to take any more antibiotics for her recurrent chest infections.

A fundamental principle of medical practice, dating from the time of Hippocrates, is that doctors must act in the best interests of their patients. This duty involves balancing respect for the patient's autonomy with a paternalistic approach to their care, which raises questions about the nature of autonomy and paternalism. The next section will deal with these questions.

What is autonomy?

It has been said that the only thing that seems completely clear about autonomy is that it means different things to different writers. Definitions have included notions of liberty, independence, self-determination and self-knowledge. The only constant feature of these definitions is that autonomy is a characteristic of persons and that it is a desirable quality to possess.[1] The word itself derives from the Greek (*auto* meaning self and *nomy*, law) and referred originally to the right of the citizens of the independent city states in Greece to make their own laws. It is now used in relation to individuals and contrasts with 'heteronomy', which means 'moral law commanded from without'.

The concept of individual autonomy was developed by Immanuel Kant (1724–1804), who considered it to be of fundamental importance to morality. It has been claimed that he invented the conception of morality as autonomy.[2] He linked autonomy with rationality and considered that an autonomous person is motivated by purely rational principles and has a duty to express his or her autonomy.

Other philosophers have identified the importance of reason and autonomy in defining what a 'person' is. In contrast, David Hume (1711–76) considered that reason alone can never be a motive of an action or decision: 'it can never oppose passion in the direction of the will'. The importance of acknowledging the emotional, as well as the rational, components of moral judgments was emphasised by John Benson in an important essay on autonomy.[3] Gerald Dworkin acknowledged the problem posed by the different interpretations of autonomy and attempted to develop a theory of autonomy. For example, he looked at wishes or desires and distinguished between first- and second-order desires. We, as individuals, may want to have another cigarette or eat another chocolate bar (this is our first-order desire), but we may also want to stop smoking or lose weight (our second-order desire), because we know that smoking and being overweight are bad for our health. Dworkin and other philosophers hold that autonomous persons can reflect critically on their first-order desires and have the capacity to accept or attempt to change these in the light of their second-order desires.

> By exercising such a capacity, persons define their nature, give meaning and coherence to their lives and take responsibility for the kind of person they are.[4]

Autonomy has been developed and expanded by bioethicists, including Professor Ranaan Gillon, a philosopher and GP.[5] He has defined autonomy as 'the capacity to think, decide and act (on the basis of such thought and decision) freely and independently'. This definition emphasises two aspects of autonomy:

- the capacity or ability of the autonomous person to make independent decisions and to act on those decisions
- the freedom to act autonomously, although limits must be imposed on an individual's autonomy when it impinges on the autonomy of another person.

Autonomy has been described as a spectrum or continuum and this is a useful concept in the context of healthcare, as we shall see later. At one end of the spectrum is negative autonomy or freedom from interference, which is an anti-paternalistic approach and at the other end is positive autonomy or the enablement of autonomy. Autonomy here is interpreted as liberty, and extends Isaiah Berlin's concept of positive and negative liberty. John Stuart Mill (1806–73) wrote a lot about the liberty of the individual as 'the free development of individuality ... one of the leading essentials of well being', although he rarely used the term 'autonomy'.[6]

Who is autonomous?

Before we look at autonomy and paternalism in the context of everyday general practice, we need to consider the attributes of an autonomous individual, which is particularly important when decisions involve children, individuals with learning disability, the mentally ill and the elderly (*see* Chapter 10). As we have seen, Kant considered that the ability to reason was the fundamental attribute of the autonomous person, which raises the question as to what degree of rationality a person must demonstrate in order to be considered autonomous and whether this can be assessed. An autonomous action has been defined as:

- intentional
- when the individual has understood all the choices
- free of controlling influences.[7]

As we shall see later, these aspects reflect the legal definition of a person's capacity to give consent to treatment.

In healthcare, autonomy is highly valued and the autonomous person is seen as rational and independent. If this is so, does it imply that dependency and those who are dependent are seen as having less value? Campbell believes not and argues that autonomy does not carry *intrinsic* moral value. He also considers the potentially negative impact on the vulnerable of emphasising autonomy as independence.[8] This has also been raised by Agich, who has written extensively on autonomy in the context of those who need long-term care. He believes that respecting the autonomy of vulnerable people, for example the elderly, 'requires attending to those things that are truly and significantly meaningful and important for elders'.[9]

Autonomy can be considered as a spectrum or continuum in another way. A person's ability to exercise his autonomy will change during his lifetime. The capacity to reason and make independent choices is not present during early childhood, and may be impaired at the end of life. Illness may impair the ability of a person to exercise their autonomy, which will be restored when the person returns to health. Campbell sees the autonomous, independent individual as a 'mere philosopher's abstraction' as we all have periods of appropriate dependence which may be 'the precursor to a restoration of autonomy'.[10]

Other factors, such as culture and age, will influence a person's desire and ability to exercise their autonomy. We all recognise that an older person is more likely than someone in their twenties to say 'You decide, doctor'.

What is paternalism?

The paternalistic approach to healthcare mirrors the relationship between father and child; the father has the best interests of the child at heart and is guided by these when making decisions on the child's behalf. Paternalism has been defined by as 'The interference with a person's liberty of action, justified by reasons referring exclusively to the welfare, good, happiness, needs, interest or values of the person being coerced.'[11] In other words we act paternalistically when we believe that our action is in the person's best interests and justify it in that way. Many would object to the use of the word 'coerced' in the context of the doctor–patient relationship. That is certainly true if it means forcing a patient to make a decision against their will, but it is important to remember that there are subtle forms of coercion, for example the way in which information is presented to a person.

The paternalistic or 'doctor knows best' approach to medical care has predominated until fairly recently. Its origins lay in the rise of scientific medicine and the consequent imbalance of power between doctor and patient. The doctor's power was invested in his knowledge of the causes and treatment of disease, which were considered to be the key, and only, factors in deciding how a patient's problem should be managed. In addition, patients were considered incapable of understanding medicine and in need of protection from the truth about their illness. But this is changing with the recognition that patients have their own expert knowledge about their condition, that their preferences and values are part of the decision-making process and that involving them in their care leads to better health outcomes.[12]

Paternalism does have a place in caring for patients in general practice[13] and we shall see this in the discussion of the cases. One of the extreme examples of appropriate paternalism is the admission of a person to hospital under the Mental Health Act 1983. Personal autonomy is overridden by the concern for the patient's safety and that of other people. However there is always a risk that paternalism will encourage patients to be the passive recipients of healthcare and not to take appropriate responsibility for their own health.

Respect for autonomy

The major philosophers have emphasised that we have a moral obligation to respect the autonomy of others. Kant expressed this in his moral imperative, which says that we should treat others as ends and not as the means to ends. Mill saw respect for the autonomy of others as essential in promoting the happiness and wellbeing of the majority.

Respect for a patient's autonomy has been identified as one of the four ethical principles by Beauchamp and Childress.[14] The other principles are beneficence (the obligation to benefit the patient, to act in their best interest), non-maleficence (the obligation to avoid causing harm) and justice (fairness in the distribution of risks and benefits). Many have found the four-principle approach to analysing and resolving ethical dilemmas in healthcare very helpful. The principles are *prima facie* – that is they can be overridden by competing moral considerations. Respect for autonomy is now considered by many to trump the other principles, with Ranaan Gillon saying that respect for autonomy should be 'first among equals'.[15] Others are critical of the principled approach to ethical dilemmas.[16] There are certainly problems with the approach, particularly when, for example, autonomy conflicts with the principles of beneficence and non-maleficence, as we shall see later in this chapter.

Do we have a right to have our autonomy respected? The concept of rights is complex and is discussed in Chapter 4. In the context of autonomy, we have a qualified right (that is it can be overridden by other considerations) but not an absolute moral or legal right to have our autonomy respected. Respect for a person's autonomy must involve respect for the autonomy of others. For example, a patient's right to confidentiality or to receive a specific form of care can be overridden by consideration of the public good. Correspondingly, doctors have an absolute duty to respect a person's right to healthcare but not to their demands for a particular form of care, as we shall see later in the case of Ms C.

Balancing autonomy and paternalism

There is no doubt that the pendulum has swung from paternalistic care towards respect for a person's autonomy. A number of factors have influenced this movement.

The socio-political climate

Within the NHS, the Patients' Charter was introduced in the UK in 1992 and laid down the 'rights' to which every patient was entitled. Although the Charter was welcomed by many, it was also criticised for placing insufficient emphasis on the responsibilities of patients.

The law

In 1948, the Universal Declaration of Human Rights introduced the current emphasis on autonomy and rights. This led to the European Convention on Human Rights, which was incorporated into English law in the Human Rights Act of 1998. Respect for a person's autonomy is reflected in several articles of the Act: for example, the right to life (article 2), the right to respect for private and family life (article 8), freedom of thought, conscience and religion (article 9) and freedom of expression (article 10).[17]

Professional practice and accountability

The inquiry into the inadequacy of the paediatric cardiac surgery service in Bristol highlighted the need for change in the way doctors interact with patients.[18] Many of the recommendations made by the inquiry focused on the need for better, more open communication between doctors and their patients (or their parents). Patients need to be more involved in decisions about their care and to be given adequate information when asked to consent to treatment. The General Medical Council (GMC) has stated that one of the duties of doctors is to 'respect the right of patients to be fully involved in decisions about their care'.[19]

Evidence-based medicine

The evidence-based 'movement' of the 1990s stressed the importance of basing clinical decisions on sound scientific evidence rather than the authority of the doctor, suggesting a move away from paternalism.

But the original definition of evidence-based medicine still had a paternalistic approach to healthcare.

> The conscientious, explicit and judicious use of current best evidence in making decisions about the care of individual patients.[20]

This definition was criticised by many and subsequently the importance of taking into account a patient's values and preferences was recognised and the term 'evidence-based patient choice' was coined.[21]

Research studies

A number of studies have found that the majority of patients want to be more involved in their care and that the opportunity to choose leads to greater satisfaction and better health outcomes. Some of these studies have been described and discussed in a recent book by Angela Coulter, who argues strongly that paternalism has had its day and that the patient's role must be redefined to emphasise their autonomy.[22]

From theory to practice

The doctor–patient relationship is at the heart of effective healthcare. It is where the balance between paternalism and respect for the autonomy of the patient presents opportunities and challenges, and this is particularly so in primary care because of its unique features. Primary care physicians deal with patients with undifferentiated illness, they usually have continuity of care, deal with acute and chronic illness and, in the UK and other countries, are the gateway to secondary care. In addition, prevention of disease and health promotion are both important parts of a primary care physician's role and emphasise their role in managing resources and their responsibility to their practice population as well as to individual patients.

Studies of consultations in general practice have led to the development of models of clinical decision-making and three styles can be identified:[23]

- the paternalistic approach when the doctor decides and the patient consents
- shared decision-making
- the patient decides after receiving the information.

Sharing of the decision-making process reflects patient-centred care that involves being responsive to a patient's wants, needs and preferences. It also implies that the patient must assume mutual responsibility for the decision and its outcomes.

Respecting a patient's autonomy does not necessarily mean non-interference or acquiescing to their choice. In helping a patient to make a decision, a doctor's role is to enable them to exercise their autonomy. The first step is an acceptance of the fundamental principle that a patient has a right to be involved in their own care, although this right may be qualified by other considerations, as we shall see later. The following steps reflect the importance of good communication.

- Provide the patient with relevant information in a form they can understand, particularly the risks and benefits of an intervention.
- Try to establish how much they want to be involved in decision-making.
- Try to establish what they would like done and why.
- Understand the reasons for their decision.
- Respect that decision during their ongoing care.

Autonomy has been described as a 'slippery concept' by Wyatt, who argued that it has a clear theoretical meaning for philosophers but is elusive and difficult for those working in his own field of foetal medicine and also in intensive care units.[24] The rest of this chapter will examine the problem of putting 'respect for a person's autonomy' into practice in the context of the case scenarios. Some of the conflicts that may arise will also be explored.

Autonomy and consent

In her discussion of trust and autonomy, O'Neill has argued against the current tendency to see respect for a person's autonomy only in the context of informed consent.[25] In primary care, however, many of the issues around paternalism and respect for autonomy do arise in the context of consent to treatment. A number of the cases described earlier focus on the patient's consent to treatment. Obtaining valid consent is a legal and moral obligation placed on doctors.

The key features of valid consent are that the patient is competent and makes a voluntary, informed decision about whether or not they want to accept the treatment. It is interesting to note that these features are similar to those of autonomy, as quoted earlier. So giving or withholding consent is about a patient making an informed choice. The role of the doctor has been described as 'to determine what is in the patient's own best interests. You may wish to recommend a treatment or a course of action, but you must not put pressure on patients to accept your advice.'[26]

A potential conflict between beneficence, respect for a patient's autonomy and behaving paternalistically arises when:

- a competent patient refuses treatment for a life-threatening condition (Mrs G)
- a competent patient wants the doctor to make the decision about their treatment (Mrs E)
- there is doubt about a patient's competence to make an autonomous decision (Ms A)
- a patient is obviously not able to give consent (Ms D).

The competent patient and decisions at the end of life

Caring for dying patients presents doctors with difficult ethical and legal issues, perhaps especially for a GP who has cared for a chronically ill patient such as Mrs G over many years. If you were the clinician caring for her it would help to consider the following questions.

- Is Mrs G competent to refuse further treatment for her recurrent chest infections?
- If so, does she have a right to refuse treatment?
- Has she made a 'living will' or advance directive?
- How does her request balance with your duty to 'do good' and 'do no harm'?

Mrs G is competent to exercise her autonomy and to make decisions about her care if it can be established that she understands the implications of her refusal. If she is judged competent, then she has a moral and legal right to refuse further treatment. She may have made an advance directive, which would come into force if she was found to lack competence. An advance directive is now legally binding, assuming that it was made without external pressure when the patient was competent and it covers the circumstances of their final illness. The potential conflict for her GP lies in his or her duty to act in her best interests (beneficence) and to respect her autonomy. But it could be strongly argued that respecting her decision not to have her life prolonged, although perhaps difficult for a doctor to accept and deal with, *is* acting in her best interests.

The acceptance of a person's right to refuse treatment can be seen as a 'triumph of autonomy', but it does not extend to patients who cannot end their own lives because of physical disability. The right to die by assisted suicide was raised in the UK courts and in the European Court of Human Rights by Diane Pretty who had motor neurone disease and wanted her husband to assist her to commit suicide. The courts rejected her request, arguing that the rights of one group to exercise their autonomy could not be allowed to undermine the rights of others.[27]

The competent patient and paternalism

Mrs E wants her doctors to make decisions for her. This presents an apparent conflict between respecting her autonomy and acting paternalistically. It can be argued that agreeing to her request is a way of respecting her autonomy and to her benefit. However this must involve careful discussion to ensure that she understands all the relevant issues. Whilst overt paternalism may be appropriate for a few patients, there is evidence that it does not benefit the majority and fosters passivity and dependence on healthcare professionals.

Mrs E has also told her GP that she does not want to know the results of any further tests. Studies have shown that the majority of people want to know the facts and the 'truth' about their illness. The majority of doctors would consider that this is usually desirable and in so doing they are respecting the patient's autonomy. However, it is clearly important to consider the potential conflict between 'telling the truth' and not causing the patient harm. Once again this emphasises the importance of good communication between patient and doctor. Mrs E's reasons for not wanting to know would need careful exploration and would need to be kept under review, particularly when she entered the terminal stages of her illness.

The patient who may not be competent

Ms A has Down's syndrome and a moderate level of learning disability. She is less certain than her mother about having a hysterectomy. In considering whether or not she should have a hysterectomy, the following questions are relevant.

- Is she autonomous?
- If so, is she able to exercise her autonomy? Does she have the capacity to understand the implications of a hysterectomy and make a decision?
- If so, is she free to exercise her autonomy, for example is she free from pressure from her family and others, including her GP?

The fact that a person has a learning disability does not mean that they lack autonomy. The answer to the first question lies in Gillon's definition of autonomy and would involve an assessment of her cognitive ability. Autonomy has been described as an ability to be fostered and developed rather than something which a person possesses.[28] Hence the role of her GP is to enable Ms A to exercise her autonomy as far as possible, which would include discussing the advantages and disadvantages of hysterectomy at her level of understanding and also gaining an understanding of her needs and preferences.

The other aspect of autonomy and valid consent to treatment is that the person should be free of all controlling influences. This would be an important part of the consultation with Ms A and her mother.

The patient who is incompetent

Mrs D is unconscious because of hypoglycaemia. She is obviously not able to exercise her autonomy and give her consent to life saving treatment. Her GP is morally and legally bound to treat her under the 'doctrine of necessity'. This case demonstrates one form of fluctuating autonomy. Before she became unconscious Mrs D was a rational person, fully able to exercise her autonomy; but later she was incapable of consenting and her GP acted 'paternalistically' in her best interests. His short-term paternalism helped her to regain her autonomy.

Autonomy and prevention

Preventing disease and promoting the health of patients is becoming an increasingly important role for the practice team and is now linked to practice income. Issues relating to disease prevention may be raised by the patient or doctor during a consultation initiated by the patient. Alternatively the patient may be called to attend a special clinic devoted to chronic disease management or screening. Some have argued that this emphasis on prevention medicalises risk factors and may compromise patient autonomy.[29]

Mr B has attended such a clinic and has declined advice and help about smoking. He clearly has a right to do this and his autonomy must be respected, although this may raise conflicts for his GP. The role of his GP is to explain the risks of smoking and to do this in such a way that Mr B can exercise his autonomy – that is given the opportunity to reflect on the impact of his second-order desire (wanting to give up smoking) on his first-order desire to continue to smoke.

Mr B has also refused take the medication prescribed for him. Evidence suggests that almost half of all drugs prescribed are not taken, particularly drugs such as statins prescribed to prevent disease. We no longer say that Mr B is 'non-compliant' or 'non-adherent'. The abandoning of terms 'compliance' and 'adherence' in favour of 'concordance' reflects changes in the balance between autonomy and paternalism in the consultation. Compliance involves following the advice and rules set by the doctor; concordance involves shared decision-making.[30]

Autonomy and the public good

We have said that respecting the autonomy of an individual is not an absolute duty for a doctor and consideration must be given to the autonomy of others and to the good of the public. Ms C has refused a hospital delivery and insists that she has a 'right' to a home birth. But does she? The answer is that she has neither a moral nor a legal right to a home birth. Two things are clear: first, exercising her autonomy does not mean demanding treatment and second, respecting her autonomy does not mean meeting her demands. The needs of other people must be considered, for example, in her area there may be a shortage of midwives and, by agreeing to her demands, the service for other women may be impaired.

Ms C's history of a previous complicated delivery and the increased risks in this pregnancy raise the issue of whether or not the rights of the fetus should be considered. Although the fetus has no rights in law, it is inevitable that the wellbeing of the fetus should be considered in discussions between Ms C and those caring for her.

Although Ms C does not have a right to demand a home birth, she does have a legal right to have access to her practice records under the Data Protection Act 1998. This is a good example of the move from paternalism to respect for autonomy, which, it could be argued, is for the good of both the individual and society.

There are other examples of situations when respect for a person's autonomy may conflict with the good of the public. Some relate to the allocation of limited financial resources including the prescribing of expensive drugs. A GP has a duty to his whole practice population and the prescribing of, for example, assisted conception drugs to a few couples may limit the prescribing of a lower-cost drug to a larger number of patients. Others relate to the protection of the public. For example, a person with tuberculosis may be forced against their will to have treatment under the Public Health (Control of Disease) Act 1984.

And finally

Autonomy is a difficult concept to understand fully and respecting a person's autonomy not always easy to put into practice. This chapter began with emphasising the duty of every clinician to act in the best interests of their patient. Evidence suggests that this will usually mean respecting their autonomy and involving them in their own care. Occasionally it will mean acting paternalistically. Which is done will depend on the circumstances and knowledge of the patient. It is important to see autonomy as a dynamic concept that is context-dependent and varies through life. Our role as clinicians is to help patients to develop and exercise their autonomy, to see the consultation as a partnership between doctor and patient with a mutual respect for each other's autonomy.

Throughout this chapter the emphasis has been on autonomy as the right of the rational individual to independence or self-determination, reflecting the current socio-political climate. Questions are now being asked if this increasing emphasis on individual autonomy is harming the doctor–patient relationship and the needs of society.[31]

> No Man is an Island, entire of itself; every man is a piece of a Continent, a part of the main.
>
> John Donne

References

1 Dworkin G. *The Theory and Practice of Autonomy*. Cambridge: Cambridge University Press; 1988.
2 Schneewind JB. *The Invention of Autonomy: a history of modern moral philosophy*. Cambridge: Cambridge University Press; 1998.
3 Benson J. Who is autonomous man? *Philosophy*. 1983; **58**: 5–17.
4 *Ibid*. note 1.
5 Gillon R. *Philosophical Medical Ethics*. Chichester: John Wiley and Sons; 1994; Gillon R. Medical ethics: four principles plus attention to scope. *BMJ*. 1994; **309**: 184–8.
6 Mill JS. On liberty. In: Collini S, ed. *On Liberty*. Cambridge: Cambridge University Press; 1989.
7 Beauchamp TL, Childress J. *Principles of Biomedical Ethics*. Oxford: Oxford University Press; 2001. p. 59.
8 Campbell A. Dependency revisited. The limits of autonomy in medical ethics. In: Fulford KGW, Gillette G, Soskice JM, eds. *Medicine and Moral Reasoning*. Cambridge: Cambridge University Press; 1994.
9 Agich GJ. *Autonomy and Long-Term Care*. Oxford: Oxford University Press; 1993. p. 113.
10 *Ibid*. note 8.
11 Dworkin G. Quoted in: McKinstry B. Paternalism and the doctor–patient relationship in general practice. *BJGP*. 1992; **42**: 340–2.
12 Griffin SJ, Kinmonth AL, Veltman MWM *et al*. Effect on health-related outcomes of interventions to alter the interaction between patients and practitioners: a systematic review of trials. *Annals of Fam Med*. 2004: **2**(6): 595–608.
13 McKinstry B. Paternalism and the doctor–patient relationship in general practice. *BJGP*. 1992; **42**: 340–2.
14 *Ibid*. note 9.
15 Gillon R. Ethics needs principles – four can encompass the rest – and respect for autonomy should be 'first among equals'. *J Med Ethics*. 2003; **29**: 307–12.

16 Harris J. In praise of unprincipled ethics. *J Med Ethics*. 2003; **29**: 303–6.

17 British Medical Association. *The Impact of the Human Rights Act 1998 on Medical Decision-Making*. London: BMA; 2000.

18 The Bristol Royal Infirmary Inquiry: http://www.bristol-inquiry.org.uk/index.htm

19 General Medical Council. *Duties of a Doctor*. http://www.gmcuk.org/standards/standards_frameset.htm. 1995.

20 Sackett D, Rosenberg W. EMB: what it is and what it isn't. *BMJ*. 1996; **312**: 71–2.

21 Edwards A, Elwyn G. *Evidence-based Patient Choice*. Oxford: Oxford University Press; 2001.

22 Coulter A. *The Autonomous Patient. Ending paternalism in medical care*. London: Nuffield Trust; 2002.

23 Emanuel EJ, Emanuel LL. Four models of the physician-patient relationship. *JAMA*. 1992; **267**: 2221–6.

24 Wyatt J. Medical paternalism and the fetus. *J Med Ethics*. 2001; **27**: 15–20.

25 O'Neill O. *Autonomy and Trust in Bioethics*. Cambridge: Cambridge University Press; 2002.

26 *Ibid*. note 21.

27 Freeman MDA. Denying death its dominion: thoughts on the Diane Pretty case. *Med Law Rev*. 2002; **10**(3): 245.

28 Toon PD. *Towards a Philosophy of General Practice: a study of the virtuous practitioner* (RCGP Occasional Paper 78). London: Royal College of General Practitioners; 1999. p. 17.

29 Heath I. Who needs healthcare – the well or the sick? *BMJ*. 2005; **330**: 954–6.

30 Elwyn G, Edwards A, Britten N. 'Doing prescribing': how doctors can be more effective. *BMJ*. 2003; **327**: 864–7.

31 Stirrat GM, Gill R. Autonomy in medical ethics after O'Neill. *J Med Ethics*. 2005; **31**: 127–30.

Further reading

British Medical Association. *Medical Ethics Today*. London: BMJ Publishing; 2004.

Hope T, Savulescu J, Hendrick J. *Medical Ethics and Law*. Edinburgh: Elsevier Churchill Livingstone; 2003.

Schneider CE. *The Practice of Autonomy*. Oxford: Oxford University Press; 1998.

Chapter 3

'But it's not my fault!' Are we responsible for our health?

John Spicer

> Nothing is sure, nothing is certain, nothing is risk free, nothing is fully covered, nothing is forever. It is a noble calling, go out into the world, he would say, and do your duty.[1]
>
> William Boyd

Introduction

Although William Boyd was writing of loss adjusters and their trade, rather than of primary healthcare practitioners, there are some obvious similarities. Both deal in risk and its modification. Both deal in the interpretation of responsibilities for events – events, moreover, which include the illnesses from which we suffer and are at least in part the product of our own actions. We are, by example and according to historic doggerel, what we eat.[2] We are also what we do, what we don't do, and what we spring from. It further needs to be acknowledged that we are also none of those things, that in some part the illnesses from which we suffer are just the product of poor luck.

Epidemiology teaches us, however, that nutrition is not the only observable determinant of health: smoking status, genetic loading, housing, socio-economic status and many other factors also have an impact on health. Any or all of these influences are modifiable by an individual's own behaviour, as well as by clinical intervention.

In primary care, clinicians are faced with the task of advising individuals about the generation and treatment of illnesses that arise, among other factors, out of their behaviour. A consideration of the interrelation between those illnesses and autonomous individual behaviour seems therefore apposite, and that will form the basis for this chapter. I will be taking the meaning of the word 'illness' in its established sense: that of a biological process causing human suffering, which may lead to the seeking of professional help.[3] I will also consider briefly how some of these themes may affect resource allocation decisions in healthcare.

The autonomous smoker

To begin with, consider the following case summary of a 'generic' patient, one that might present to any member of a primary healthcare team for care. For no particular reason he is named 'Bill', though he could be female, and no gender specificity is implied.

Bill

- male, aged 55
- smoker
- obesity body mass index 34
- documented hypertensive for five years
- proven single vessel coronary artery disease
- symptomatic angina pectoris on effort
- hyperlipidaemia
- inert of exercise
- father died of myocardial infarction, aged 60
- three teenage children
- plumber
- impaired glucose tolerance

This is a rather bald statement of mainly physiological descriptors attaching to Bill. Perhaps there is even an implied criticism of lifestyle inherent in the summary. Almost all of the descriptors include an aspect of aetiology referable to behaviour prior to his illness: he has smoked, rarely exercised and possibly eaten 'unhealthily'. A fuller narrative more representative of that gleaned over time by members of a primary care team could run as follows.

Bill was born into a family of four in the early 1950s. He attended the local secondary modern school, leaving without exam success, but was apprenticed into the plumbing and heating trade. He found this to his liking and progressed well.

His father died suddenly when Bill was 15, leaving him without another male in the house and markedly bereaved for some years. Relationships with his sister and mother were good.

He fell in with minor criminality in his late teens, gathering a conviction for burglary. This seemed to have had a profound effect upon

Continued

him as thereafter he threw himself into his work, eventually forming his own business aged 25. He now employs two other people and
has a constant run of work, being highly valued by his customers.

His wife Barbara works part-time in the business and they have a
long-term and happy marriage. Her health has only been marred by
a short depressive period some years ago at around the time Bill had
an affair with his secretary.

Such a narrative may *only* emerge over the course of a long-standing relationship with Bill and his family. Whilst the first summary more closely
resembles that gained in the out-patient clinic of a hospital, the second
description seems more attuned to that revealed and reviewed by primary
healthcare team members in their conversations with the patient. A number of questions are suggested by such histories, including, for example,
the following.

- How should healthcare professionals regard Bill?
- Should they dispassionately regard him as the victim of pathological
  processes beyond his control that require their intervention in his
  assistance?
- Should they consider him responsible for his current state by virtue of
  his past behaviour and thus less deserving of their professional efforts?
- What is the nature of the moral duty, as a member of a caring profession, in offering Bill the best treatment for his 'illness'.

The questions are suggested because management of the illness depends
at least partially on modification of his behaviour: his coronary artery
disease and its ensuing symptoms are unlikely to improve without smoking cessation. Implicit in this empirically observed biological fact is the
corollary that coronary heart disease is largely caused by smoking tobacco. Because Bill has smoked *inter alia*, he is ill: and if he ceases to smoke
he will have a chance of not being so. The responsibility for his fate lies
in his hands. Indeed in one analysis, implicit in the taking of such a
responsibility for past actions is a 'rectificatory or reformative' aspect to
future conduct.[4]

Another way of ascribing responsibility to Bill for his plight, or at least
that element of it referable to his smoking pattern, is to incorporate the
notion of volition. To put it differently, his voluntary decision to smoke
might lead to the ascription of responsibility for his illness. That might
seem to be quite a large step to take for several reasons.

First, it may be that Bill never knew that smoking was associated with
the negative health consequences now known to be so. In this sense,

his elective decision to smoke over many years was not necessarily autonomous, undermined as it was by a lack of information as to the consequences. Knowledge of this sort has been in the public domain for 40 years or more,[5] so it could be said to be unlikely that Bill might have been in ignorance of the consequences of what he was doing.

Second, the smoking of cigarettes is a behaviour described as addictive or in some sense compelled, perhaps as a result of the pharmacological constituents therein. So when smoking is started, there is an intrinsic, driven and almost unavoidable urge to continue that also undermines Bill's voluntary choices.

Third, his smoking may have started in his teenage years when arguably his capacity to make mature and informed choices about his behaviour was somehow less than had he been older. The bioethicist, John Harris describes these and other aspects in some detail.[6]

Modern Western clinical ethics accords greatest importance to the principle of respect for personal autonomy. As is well known, this principle is usually elevated to the status of predominance when balanced against others in the resolution of moral dilemmas in healthcare.

It is not really contentious that this is so any longer, despite its variation around the world, and this notion is at one with a diminution of paternalist clinical practice. The law and its moral footings uphold the rights of people to determine their own clinical futures. However, it should be noted that the vast literature on consent now available deals for the most part with prospective decisions by patients. That such decisions should be informed, capacitous, uncoerced and dynamic is axiomatic in the early 21st century. Indeed in this way they should be freely autonomous and thus unfettered by any of Harris' limitations.[7]

These criteria seem to have a more limited application as a retrospective tool: in allocating a personal responsibility to Bill for the outcome of his years of tobacco use, what is actually being done is interpreting the philosophical foundations of a prospective notion of consent and applying it to a personal history. Clearly this is quite a challenging logical leap to take. If nothing else, it is reminiscent of legal attribution of guilt by causation. Consider this example: if I drive my white van at high speed down a road and kill a child at a bus queue, I am guilty of a crime. I may well undergo due process and suffer punishment as a result. All other things being equal, the allocation of responsibility is clear. But if I smoke for many years, even if in a fully autonomous fashion, and then develop a smoking-related disease as Bill has done: am I quite so guilty? Is there a comparable chain of causation between the two cases? Self-evidently in the former, the death of the child has been brought about by the action of the van driver alone (as described), whereas the development of a smoking-related disease is the product of many factors interacting together, such as those listed at the head of this section. Even if many factors coalesce together as in Bill's unfortunate history, the outcome may not be negative.

Eat well, get lucky

The ethical analysis of Bill's dietary predicament is slightly more complex. In contrast with the case of smoking, in which any indulgence may be held to be harmful, food and sustenance are necessary to human flourishing. We may, quite clearly, take food in excess and render ourselves harm, or we may take an excess of one food over another, achieving the same end. In the developed world at least, inadequate access to food is not a particular problem, but rather it's over access. This chapter began with the 'we are what we eat' observation, which might be modified into 'we would like to be what we should eat'. This assumes, of course, that we would not wish to be ill as a consequence of following a 'poor' diet.

Celebrated French gastronomy[8] may have something to offer the benighted Anglo-Saxon diet in this regard. The epidemic of ischaemic heart disease (IHD) appears to affect French and Southern Mediterranean populations less: had Bill lived in Toulon rather than Manchester, for the sake of argument, he might have eaten a slightly healthier diet, taken *in toto,* and thus had less risk of IHD. Perhaps, it highlights a fourth way in which the responsibility for illness is diffused: by the conformance with locally defined patterns of behaviour, in this case dietary, which confer better health outcomes. This is not simply a matter of holding to social norms, although it is that too.

There are more complex processes at work here: it is known that people of lower socio-economic status have poorer health outcomes generally.[9] Whether this is purely dietary, or, more plausibly, the combination of many factors as already described, need not detain us. But it seems that being poor means being of poorer health and thus a powerful argument against allocation of a strict responsibility for health outcomes in the case of social disadvantage. To be poor and healthy would require more of those people than to be rich and healthy, an aspect that could be held to be inequitable.

In any event, the mechanism through which diet influences mortality seems to be within lipid metabolism, such that good empirical evidence exists showing that where individuals maintain high blood cholesterol, harm to the vascular tree can eventuate. To some extent the cholesterol level is modifiable by behaviour, as in the Mediterranean diet above, but to some extent it is not. It has been suggested that mass dietary change with or without mass medication with lipid lowering drugs might significantly reduce rates of IHD.[10] Perhaps such an intervention would have prevented Bill's illnesses. The danger, of which much has been written, is the medicalisation of everyday life.[11, 12] The risk or benefits of dietary or pharmacological intervention based on measurement of blood lipids are still unclear and argued at the margins, though clear when established. A morally strong justification to intervene on this basis appears weak in consequence.

A question that hovers around this issue is whether patients such as Bill, who 'suffer' from hyperlipidaemia, are indeed ill. In the terms described above the answer would be in the negative. But he clearly suffers with angina, at least partially related to his lipid status, and any reasonable formulation of management would include attention to an abnormal value. It seems an implausible step to accord responsibility to him to reduce his lipids on his own efforts, alone or in tandem with a lipid-lowering drug. Were he not symptomatic, but the possessor of a seriously adverse lipid profile it might be considered only a question of luck that it was so.

The precise combination of genetic and behavioural factors need not detain us in an ethical discussion, suffice to say that there are both, but it helps to gain an ethical purchase on Bill's responsibility for his illness by considering his family history. His father, for example, is recorded as dying a relatively early cardiac death. Clearly, we cannot choose our parents and therefore the genetic predispositions they bequeath us are unavoidable. It seems to be a matter of luck that Bill has the family history he has when he cannot be causally responsible for it. But as we have seen, to have that family history has an effect on his own illness pattern, as it interacts with the other factors in which he does have a certain control. If there is a moral analysis to be made of Bill's actions in smoking, eating to excess and inertia, is there an additional element of luck in the responsibility for his family history?

Consider, as Thomas Nagel does, the driver of (another) white van, who, rushing down the road to his next appointment, crosses a red light on a traffic junction and narrowly misses injuring yet another school child on his way home. Luckily the child survives in the presence of a clearly unlawful action (if not immoral): the outcome is not adverse but it could have been. If it had been, the driver would obviously have been held liable. Nagel holds that: 'where a significant aspect of what someone does depends on factors beyond his control, yet we continue to treat him in that aspect as an object of moral judgement, it can be called moral luck'.[13]

The implication for Bill is that we hold his risk behaviour up as a moral enterprise. It is not morally neutral to smoke, drink to excess and overeat since the consequences may be adverse, though he may encounter good moral luck in avoiding such consequences. In the case of poor moral luck, or adverse consequences, we may judge it, as Nagel has, 'moral determination by the actual',[14] or what is known more usually as strict, responsibility.

What are the implications of ascription of 'strict' responsibility[15] to Bill's health-related behaviour? Arguably it might lead to withdrawal of access to treatment, which could have implications for his current symptoms such as they are and considerable impact on his future life expectancy. It may lead to a change in the way his health advisors regard him.

Jonathan Glover[16] has analysed responsibility into four areas, which may lead to blame, praise, reward or punishment. If a decision is made to withdraw treatment from Bill because his clinical condition is self-induced, it seems that he is being blamed and perhaps punished for it. There might be arguments in favour of this. Others might be induced to avoid such behaviour with subsequent improvements in public health, for example. His early demise would open the door for healthcare spending on more 'deserving' cases whom we might not wish to blame or punish.

As a moral enterprise, Bill's behaviour affects not only himself, but also others. Given his illness, there are implications for his family and the other people around him. Their lives are inevitably changed, perhaps for the worse, by the situation in which he and they find themselves. More broadly, as Bill claims a share of healthcare resources consequent upon his illness, others are limited in their choices as a result.

But consider the meaning of 'responsibility' a little further. For George Agich,[17] despite its being a 'richly ambiguous and complex concept', responsibility in strict terms is essentially a notion of accountability that ethically demands understanding, deliberative abilities, knowledge and decision-making. This reflective and critical dimension to responsibility is echoed in the work of William Glannon.[18]

It is similar, but not identical, to Harris' discussion of autonomous thinking.[19] In Bill's case, if assumptions are to be made about his responsibility for his illnesses, Agich might demand that he is demonstrably in possession of full knowledge and understanding as to the genesis of such problems, as well as being in a position to weigh up opinions on both sides of an empirical argument. To which we might add that Bill should know the consequences of his illness to his family and the wider community too.

More than anything else, if Bill is to be judged ethically, he must be considered free to make such decisions with respect to smoking and eating, continually and constantly. It must be doubted whether in reality this can be so.

To some extent it is more plausible to argue against strict responsibility for actions in the sense which it is being discussed *a propos* of Bill by consideration of character. His character,[20] however described, is moulded by innate (or nature) determinants and experiences (or nurture) determinants. The expression in behavioural terms of our genes is not, as Donna Dickenson notes, automatic: our characters as individuals must be determined by other factors as well. The narratives of our lives and our relationships with others are examples she quotes.[21]

The latter are sketchily outlined in the second, more narrative, description of Bill. In that sense, the more voluntary aspects of Bill's plight as summarised in the first description are not all ascribable to the events (among others) in the second. This is not to offer a determinist hostage to fortune and accept that events could not have turned out differently for Bill: life is clearly too complex for that. Rather it might augment the argument from autonomy that is it implausible for healthcare professionals to 'blame' Bill for his illnesses and 'punish' him with diminished treatment as a result.

But I might die?

It is apparent that Bill, looked at from the perspective of potentially positivist healthcare professionals, is at risk of death, at least prematurely, if not imminently. Of course, patients such as Bill can cheat their risk analysis and survive unexpectedly, but population statistics do not support this state of affairs.

Where death may be imminent by virtue of patients' own behaviour, as in the cases of suicidal patients, doctors and others lie under a duty to intervene where there is a mental illness 'state'. Such an intervention may include paternalistic clinical decision-making. Ethical justifications for such actions have been advanced[22] and rejected.[23]

One way of interpreting Bill's continuing adverse health behaviour is that he is bringing forward the time of his death and that if he should continue to eat unhealthily, smoke and be immoderate in alcohol, he is knowingly approaching, if not actually seeking, death. He may not intend an early death, but it is certainly foreseeable, by reference to empirical evidence as already described.

So does a distinction between the imminent suicide of a mentally disturbed patient and the slow unsought demise of a patient like Bill rest on an arguable distinction between foreseeabililty and intentionality?

At first sight, this seems an unlikely prospect: few healthcare professionals would agree that the patients they see of Bill's type actually intend to die as a result of their behaviour, yet much of the clinical task is to clarify the foreseeable nature of the problems and bring about autonomous, positive choices in their behaviour.

It is possible to be fairly sure about the nature of the risk facing Bill. It is less sure where the risks, of whatever origin, are preclinical. Helping patients to foresee their risks might be held to be potentially burdensome in itself because they might, in a neat echo of Glover, develop guilt and self-blame.[24] Nonetheless, it is generally held that good clinical practice in this era should be patient-centred, one aspect of which is that responsibility in health outcome is handed back to, or at the very least shared with, the patient. The justification for this ethically is the avoidance of paternalist practice, wherein decisions are taken for, rather than by, the patient.[25]

So Bill may not intend an early death, but, if he is fully informed, he in a position to foresee it. The behaviours he might change to achieve a positive outcome are then limited by his will. That the will may be constrained in some way implies lack of freedom of the will, a state roughly analogous in this area to addiction.

Harris[26] regards addiction as a limiting factor on autonomous decision-making and if we regard Bill as addicted to tobacco or indeed any other aspect of his personal behaviour, then it follows that responsibility for the consequences of such must inevitably be reduced. Philosophically, what is being described is indeed a determinist approach to the interpretation of his behaviour: it could not have been or would be less likely to be any other than what it was. There seem to be two issues at variance here.

First, if we regard addiction as an illness in its own right, then a conception of Bill's 'addictive' behaviour merits 'treatment' as an adjunct to whatever other treatment he might require for the physical manifestations of that addiction.

Or, on the other hand, if we regard addiction as merely a weakness of the will, then strict responsibility is plausibly allocated. Again, modern clinical practice would lend weight to the argument that addictions, including tobacco addiction, are illnesses meriting intervention. Public policy, as exemplified by the UK government actions in recent years, has sharply increased resources into smoking cessation in primary care on the utilitarian justification of reduced harms, but also tacitly acknowledges the construction of addiction as illness.

It is unlikely that Bill intends to die an early death, even if his healthcare advisors foresee it and even if he himself foresees it on accepting their information. An ethical case for a paternalist or coercive treatment regime, in the manner of a mentally disturbed and suicidal patient, is not made;

and the distinction rests not on foreseeability and intention, but rather on the differences in autonomous function.

The professional view

Earlier in this chapter a question was asked, and temporarily unanswered, about the regard with which a putative healthcare professional should show Bill. This question takes in a number of themes that merit further thought. Might there be differences between the regard which ordinary citizens and clinicians show him? Clearly lay and professional people are separated at least by a degree of duty to him.[27]

Professional regulatory bodies are quite firm about the fact that there should be no differences in care for people whose illnesses are self-inflicted or of 'lifestyle'. The Health Professions Council, an umbrella body regulating healthcare professionals, requires its members not to: 'allow your views about patients [...] sex, age, colour, race, disability, sexuality, social or economic status, lifestyle, culture, or religious beliefs to affect the way you treat them or the professional advice you give'.[28]

The General Medical Council (GMC), regulating doctors, applies similar language but adds 'you must not refuse or delay treatment because you believe that patients' actions have contributed to their condition.'[29]

A slightly different slant on this issue is revealed by the Nursing and Midwifery Council: 'You are personally accountable for ensuring that you promote and protect the interests and dignity of patients and clients, irrespective of gender, age, race, ability, sexuality, economic status, lifestyle, culture and religious or political beliefs.'[30]

These examples, despite their minor differences of emphasis, illustrate the professional standards operating in the UK. Comparable standards exist elsewhere. Thus healthcare professionals are required to treat Bill in the same fashion whether or not it might be held that his illness is in some way self-inflicted. Primary care practitioners of all types cannot avoid these professional bodies' rules: although an interesting discussion might be had as to the source of moral authority in these statutory or self-regulating agencies.

But, as the commentator Anja has it, the first obligation of any healthcare professional in regarding a person with morbid obesity, as Bill has, is to understand, to see the world from that perspective, to be empathetic. And furthermore, not to regard such a person as 'irresponsible, immature, hedonic, undisciplined, sickly, defiant, and morally disgusting',[31] as might be commonly thought. As far as that goes, it is not, by generally accepted custom, contentious. For the most part, it seems plausible to assume that conceptions of human suffering as exemplified by Bill are common between healthcare professionals and others. He is, after all, an individual in need. Differences, or at least surprising manifestations of public views, may exist in populations of people like Bill.

There is some evidence that, at least in terms of allocation of public resources to health, there is some partiality of view. One report from the US suggested that the public would preferentially allocate organs for transplants to non-smokers, non-alcoholics and non-drug misusers on the grounds of self-induced organ failure.[32] Similar reports abound.[33]

Clearly what is suggested by these studies is that a public view exists that patients who have some 'responsibility' for their illnesses should be treated less equally that those who do not. They are less deserving of treatment, perhaps because of the attributes that Anja refers to.[34] Historically, it seems that these views became prominent in the 1970s, showing marked changes from hitherto.[35]

This disconnection may be due to differences in the public's view of individuals, to whom it is easier to attach an empathetic regard, and populations, where it might not be so. It may also be associated with a popular interpretation of *desert*: that to some extent, people should get what they deserve in terms of their health risk behaviour. More usefully, perhaps, it might be suggested that what is operating here is confusion between two notions of justice.

Healthcare professionals should be more familiar with the idea of *distributive* justice, where what is at issue is the grounds on which a limited healthcare budget can be allocated to differing and deserving areas of interest. Many criteria have been advanced on how to decide such allocations, only one of which is the area of desert, which generally in the literature takes a low priority in determining a fair and equitable system. It might be added that a discussion about personal responsibility for health would only happen given an environment of scare resources, as Kantian notions of duties to self seem to generate little interest outside of narrow philosophical discourse.

Retributive justice, the arena under which punishments are handed down after due process of law, is concerned with personal responsibility for actions if nothing else. However, retributive justice is all about crime and criminal behaviour, more relevant to the errant drivers of vans, and an unlikely reference point for healthcare decision-making.[36]

We may be familiar with the descriptors of professional duty to patients like Bill as detailed at the start of this section, but the idea that there may be patients' duties is perhaps more challenging. To some extent this develops the moral notion that we all, as patients who consume scarce resources, might have duties to one another. That this might be so was raised by the president of Germany in 1997, following a round of health reforms, which withdrew, *inter alia*, citizens' access to spa treatments under the German health system.[37]

Heather Draper and Tom Sorell amplify this point more fully from the perspective of counterbalancing clinicians' and patients' duties.[38] On the grounds of duties to self and others, it is held that doctors may be released from 'captivity' as helpers. In a recent example of a new drug being associated with rare but serious adverse effects, some serious journalistic comment[39] has included the suggestion that patients, when informed, actually do bear some responsibility for the medications they take and do not automatically have a cause in action against drug manufacturers on the grounds of negligence. This would seem to run counter to previous lay discourse, which takes the notion of a new drug being approved for general use as immunity against adverse effect.

Some implications for clinical practice

Several themes have emerged thus far in this discussion, which might be usefully restated. Repeatedly, I have referred to empirical work *demonstrating* that links exist between various behaviours and negative health consequences. Broadly speaking, such studies are quantitative and derive from large populations – the meat and drink of epidemiology. From such work, risk calculations are made as to the likelihood of individual events happening and are used as a means of counselling and managing patients like Bill in primary care. This rather neat and positivist scheme of things could miss several important qualifications.

Initially one might question the application of large studies to the individual: simply to assume, for example, that the use of a statin reduces the chances of a second cardiac event by a quarter in a given population[40] and that it would thus reduce Bill's chances similarly, is a large step to take. It is part of the informed decision but no more. Bill and his healthcare professionals cannot know whether he is part of the benefited quarter or not. By extension, he cannot have a responsibility to take such a treatment, whether or not he can be accorded a responsibility for its genesis.

Part of the reason why Bill cannot know whether he will benefit from a treatment like a statin or indeed smoking cessation, prudent use of alcohol, dietary changes or the taking of exercise is his complexity as a biological system. Empirical research as it proceeds will engender more and more knowledge and greater statistical information about his disease processes, but what it will never provide is certainty as to its efficacy. Research into the application of large population studies to individuals may be better done by a qualitative methodology.[41] Healthcare professionals can offer Bill the likelihood of benefit but that is all.

In doing so, particularly in primary care, the relationships between clinicians and patients are of prime importance. They are relationships that can build up over many years (*see* Chapter 1). Suffice to say here that the notion of trust between healthcare professional and patient may help people like Bill to interpret the very complex information referred to above into a treatment plan consistent with Bill's own values, which may, or indeed may not, be compatible with 'benefit', defined in terms of statistical outcome. The trust relationship is unlikely to be at one with a notion of responsibility as blame or guilt-based on Bill's prior behaviour or, indeed, an interpretation of that behaviour as seeking his early demise as an intended, rather than foreseen, outcome. Healthcare professionals should, as Rogers argues, trust their patients too.[42]

It is also likely to be at variance with the involvement of the primary care team in rationing decisions that incorporate notions of desert. Even if some public surveys might suggest that those who, by their own actions, bring about their illnesses should be relatively disadvantaged, there seem to be no reasons why professionals should, as professionals, hold similar views. As suggested above, it might be considered an aspect of professional duty that it should be so. Anything less may, indeed, be regarded as coercive care.[43] As has been recently noted,[44] tax or health insurance policies that reward healthy lifestyle decisions in citizens and punish unhealthy lifestyles financially would not undermine relationships between patients and clinicians. The necessary corollary would be that clinicians are at one remove from policy makers. In fact, a state of tension between policy makers who may wish to distribute healthcare resources according to desert and primary care practitioners who advocate for their 'Bills' might be held to be a very good basis for creative rationing decisions. Rationing, of course, is the driver here for were it not so, questions about responsibility for health might not so readily surface.

In this chapter, I have tried to resist the perhaps tempting idea that healthcare professionals, and particularly those in primary care, should use the ascription of personal responsibility as a criterion for delivery or allocation of care. It is not a novel view[45] but one that it may become necessary to state more forcefully in the future.

References

1 Boyd W. *Armadillo*. London: Penguin; 1998.
2 And now the title of a popular volume published by a TV expert.
3 Boorse C. On the distinction between disease and illness. In: Nelson JL, Nelson HL, editors. *Meaning and Medicine: a reader in the philosophy of healthcare*. New York: Routledge; 1999.
4 Blustein J. On taking responsibility for one's past. *J App Phil*. 2000; **17**(1): 1–19.

5 Ever since *Action on Smoking and Health*, published by the RCGP in 1962, and a myriad of publications thereafter.

6 These categories are described in Harris J. *The Value of Life: an introduction to medical ethics*. London: Routledge: 1985, Ch. 10, as descriptors of autonomous behaviour.

7 Harris J. *The Value of Life: an introduction to medical ethics*. London: Routledge: 1985.

8 Burr ML. Explaining the French paradox. In: Siddell M, Jones L, Katz J, Peberdy A, editors. *Debates and Dilemmas in Promoting Health: a reader*. Basingstoke: Palgrave Macmillan; 2003. Also *J R Soc Health*. 1995; **115**(4): 217–19.

9 Lynch JW, Kaplan GA, Salonen JT. Why do poor people behave poorly? Variation in adult health behaviours and psychosocial characteristics by stages in the socio-economic lifecourse. *Soc Sci & Med*. 1997; **44**(6): 809–16.

10 Wald NJ, Law MR. A strategy to reduce cardiovascular disease by more than 80%. *BMJ*. 2003; **326**: 1419.

11 Seale C, Pattison S, Davey B, editors. *Medical Knowledge: doubt and certainty*. 2nd ed. Buckingham: Open University Press; 2001. Ch. 8.

12 Westin S, Heath I. Thresholds for normal blood pressure and serum cholesterol. *BMJ*. 2005; **330**: 1462–3.

13 Nagel T. *Moral Luck in Mortal Questions*. Cambridge: Cambridge University Press; 1979. Ch. 3.

14 *Ibid*. note 8.

15 Honoré AM. Responsibility and luck. *Law Quart Rev*. 1988; **104**: 530–3.

16 Glover J. *Responsibility*. London: Routledge and Kegan Paul; 1970.

17 Agich GJ. The concept of responsibility in medicine. In: Agich GJ, editor. *Responsibility in Health Care*. Dordrecht: Kluwer; 1982. pp. 53–73.

18 Glannon W. *The Mental Basis of Responsibility*. Aldershot: Ashgate; 2002.

19 Harris J. *Ibid*.

20 Bavidge M. *Mad or Sad?* Bristol: Bristol Classical Press; 1998. Ch. 4.

21 Dickenson D. *Risk and Luck in Medical Ethics*. Cambridge: Polity Press; 2003. Ch. 9.

22 Beauchamp TL and Childress JF. *Principles of Biomedical Ethics*. 3rd ed. Oxford: Oxford University Press; 2001.

23 Szasz T. *Law, Liberty and Psychiatry*. Syracuse: Syracuse University Press; 1989.

24 Hassed C. Taking personal responsibility for our health: nectar or poisoned chalice. *Aus Fam Physician*. 2004; **33**(1–2): 74–5.

25 May C and Mead N. Patient centeredness: a history. In: Dowrick C, Frith L, editors. *General Practice: uncertainty and responsibility*. London: Routledge; 1999. pp. 76–90.

26 Harris J. *Ibid*. note 4.

27 Gibson K. Contrasting role morality and professional morality: implications for practice. *J App Phil*. 2003; **20**(1): 17–29.

28 Health Professions Council. *Standards of Conduct, Performance and Ethics: duties as a registrant 2003*. London: Health Professions Council; 2003.

29 General Medical Council. *Good Medical Practice*. 3rd ed. London: GMC; 2001.

30 Nursing and Midwifery Council. *The NMC Code of Professional Conduct: standards for conduct, performance and ethics.* London: Nursing and Midwifery Council; 2004.

31 Anja J. Obesity, responsibility and empathy. *Case Manager.* 2004; **15**: 6.

32 Ubel P, Baron J, Asch D. Social acceptability, personal responsibility and prognosis in public judgements and transplant allocation. *Bioethics.* 1999; **13**(1): 57–68.

33 *See*, for example, Cohen C, Benjamin M. Alcoholics and liver transplantation. *JAMA.* 1991; **265**: 1299–1301 or Mechanic D. Dilemmas in rationing healthcare services: the case for implicit rationing. *BMJ.* 1995; **310**: 1655–9.

34 Anja J. *Ibid.*

35 Reiser SJ. Responsibility for personal health: a historical perspective. *J Med Phil.* 1985; **1**: 7–17.

36 For a fuller discussion of this issue, see Glover J. *Ibid.* Ch. 4.

37 Goldbeck-Wood S. Personal responsibility, not rationing is the way forward. *BMJ.* 1997; **314**: 1709.

38 Draper H and Sorell T. Patients' responsibilities in medical ethics. *Bioethics.* 2002; **16**(4): 335–52.

39 *See*, for example, Smith J. Massive payouts over Vioxx are not the answer. *The Independent*, Comment, 23.8.05.

40 Scandinavian Simvastatin Survival Study Group. Randomised trial of cholesterol lowering in 4444 patients with coronary heart disease: the Scandinavian simvastatin survival study (4S). *The Lancet.* 1994; **344**: 1383–9.

41 Slowther A, Ford S, Schofield T. Ethics of evidence based medicine in the primary care setting. *J Med Ethics.* 2004; **30**: 151–5.

42 Rogers WA. Is there a moral duty for doctors to trust their patients? *J Med Ethics.* 2002; **28**: 2.

43 Although Törbjorn Tännejö, in *Coercive Care: the ethics of choice in health and medicine.* London and New York: Routledge; 1999, does suggest an insurance premium for those who ride a bicycle without a helmet or drive a car without a safety belt.

44 Cappelen AW, Norheim OF. Responsibility in healthcare: a liberal egalitarian approach. *J Med Ethics.* 2005; **31**: 47–80.

45 Wikler D. Personal and social responsibility for health. *Ethics & International Affairs.* 2002 (Fall); **16**: 2.

Chapter 4

Human rights in primary care

Katharine Wright

> I've a right to have a second opinion.
> You've no right to talk to social services about me.
> I'm the only one who has the right to decide what's best for my child.

Introduction

When the subject of rights, and particularly 'human rights', is raised in the context of healthcare, it is very easy to focus on the more dramatic end of the spectrum, for example: experimental but risky treatment for otherwise fatal diseases or detention and compulsory treatment in secure mental health hospitals. However, while the dilemmas facing primary care practitioners may not be as headline-grabbing as those facing their colleagues working in research, mental health or intensive care, the language of rights is just as familiar in primary care as it is in other parts of the health service. For some patients, particularly those suffering from chronic and disabling conditions, there will always be more that could, potentially, be done – yet how should the needs or 'rights' of such patients be balanced against the needs or rights of others, given that all budgets are finite? If all have a 'right' to treatment, who takes priority where resources do not allow all rights to be satisfied? And what about where 'rights' appear to conflict even more directly, for example in cases of suspected child abuse or, much more commonly, where it is felt that parents are making less than wise healthcare decisions on behalf of their children? This chapter will provide a brief analysis of the difficulties raised by the language of rights and then go on to look at how the Human Rights Act 1998, which came into force in the UK on 2 October 2000, provides practical help for primary care professionals facing dilemmas of these kinds.

What do we mean by 'rights'?

The language of rights is used routinely in popular discourse. Most of us will, on a fairly regular basis, claim a right to do or possess something or, perhaps more commonly, assert that we have a right that something which might adversely affect us should *not* be done. What we will not generally do is analyse precisely what we mean when we claim these 'rights'. Do we mean that we have a *legal* right to do, or prevent, something, and that this right can, if necessary, be enforced through the courts? Or do we mean that, regardless of the state of the law in the country in which we live, we enjoy certain rights simply because we are human beings ('moral' or 'natural' rights)?

The concept of a legal right is relatively unproblematic: it is simply an expression of what the law makers in a particular country have agreed at a particular time and may be changed in accordance with the country's system for making and amending laws. However, the concept of a moral or natural right has been disputed by philosophers for centuries. At one end of the spectrum is belief in a comprehensive 'natural law', aspects of which are gradually discovered or revealed in the same way as the laws of Nature such as gravity. At the other is the belief that moral or natural rights simply do not exist and that any expression of such rights is merely a pious wish as to how we would *like* things to be in a better regulated society.[1] Moreover, even those who do believe in the concept of moral or natural rights fail to agree on the precise content of those rights or how apparently conflicting rights might be resolved. The right to be registered with a GP, for example, or the right in certain circumstances to refuse medical treatment are part of English law at the beginning of the 21st century: if these rights are not initially respected, we can take action through the courts to ensure that they are in future. However, these are not 'rights' that would necessarily be respected in another country or at another time: it is only relatively recently, for example, that English law has evolved to state clearly that a competent adult patient may refuse all treatment for physical disorders, even if that refusal leads to his or her death, and there are certainly many parts of the world where this 'right' would not be recognised. Moreover, there is far from a consensus in England that such a legal right *should* exist, with some arguing that we do not have the moral right to decide when to end our own lives.

In addition to this distinction between legal rights and moral rights, the examples above demonstrate a second distinction between what might be called 'positive' rights and 'negative' rights. In the case of a positive right or 'claim right', my right to something is matched by your duty to ensure that I receive it. An individual may only meaningfully claim to have a right to be registered with a GP if at least one GP has the duty to accept that patient onto his or her list. Negative rights, on the other hand, posit no such duty, other than a duty of non-interference by others. If I wish to exercise my right to refuse medical treatment, I am not asking anyone to undertake anything for me, other than to leave me alone. Nevertheless, an individual's claim to a negative right may still pose major ethical dilemmas for a health professional, if that professional believes that he or she is morally obliged to intervene!

This idea of negative rights has also been described as 'negative liberty' – the area within which individuals should be left alone to do or be what they want. The philosopher, Isaiah Berlin contrasts this with 'positive liberty' – the wish of the individual to be one's own master. Berlin characterises this desire thus.

> I wish, above all, to be conscious of myself as a thinking, will-ing active being, bearing responsibility for my choices and able to explain them by references to my own ideas and pur-poses. I feel free to the degree that I believe this to be true, and enslaved to the degree that I am made to realize that it is not.[2]

While Berlin is not using the language of rights, this quotation may help to elucidate much of what patients mean when they claim a right to something in the healthcare context. Many of the 'rights' claimed by patients – for example, the right to have their confidentiality respected or the right to be fully involved in decisions about their healthcare – could equally well be expressed as an assertion of their *autonomy*. While a detailed discussion of theories of autonomy is beyond the scope of this chapter,[3] the term is generally used to characterise individuals' sense of themselves as independent beings, able to make their own decisions about key aspects of their own lives (indeed, lessened in some way as human beings if they are prevented from doing so) and to accept responsibility for the consequences, good or bad, of those decisions.

So how do health professionals deal with rights?

It is clear from the brief discussion above that 'rights', at least theoret-ically, mean very different things to different people. To some, a right is only meaningful if given effect through the rule of law. Such a concept of rights would be by far the easiest to implement: if taken to its extreme, it would pose no duty on health professionals other than to ensure that their actions did not break the law. Any action which fell short of infringing the current law would therefore be acceptable (at least in the sense of not breaching anyone's rights).[4] However, the importance long placed on the need for professional ethics in areas like medicine and nursing suggests that for many such an approach is unsatisfactory and that there is a very widely held perception that health professionals should meet certain standards towards their patients regardless of the current state of the law. This claim may be expressed in terms of the rights (both positive and negative) of patients or in terms of the duties of health professionals (both to themselves and to their patients), or of both.

Yet highlighting the general belief that health professionals owe more to their patients than minimal adherence to the law does not help individual professionals deal with the dilemmas presented to them by the language of rights. If there is no agreed framework or hierarchy of rights, how can the rights claimed by patient A be evaluated or set against the conflicting rights claimed by patient B? I would suggest that there are two, linked, ways forward.

Respect for persons

A key to understanding why the notion of moral or natural rights has such a strong intuitive claim on us, despite philosophical difficulties in demonstrating their existence, is found in the quotation above from Isaiah Berlin. The idea of ourselves as 'thinking, willing active being[s], bearing responsibility for [our] choices' will be strongly endorsed by the vast majority of patients and health professionals alike. Respect for this key human trait, often summarised as 'respect for persons', is found in virtually all major moral theories, however disparate they may be in other respects. A useful tool for health professionals, when faced with the language of rights, might therefore be to consider what duties are imposed on them by respect for that patient. In some cases, the answer may seem relatively clear: 'respect for persons' will demand, for example, that the patient's confidentiality is respected; that they are treated with courtesy; that they are involved, as fully as possible, in decisions about their own care. In other cases, particularly where conflicting rights have been asserted, asking oneself what 'respect for persons' would require may seem less helpful. Since October 2000, however, a new tool has been available to health professionals to analyse and evaluate such claims: the Articles of the European Convention on Human Rights as implemented in the UK by the Human Rights Act 1998.

The European Convention and the Human Rights Act 1998

The European Convention on Human Rights was developed in the wake of the Second World War and represented an attempt to set down in an international treaty minimum standards as to how all human beings should be treated. It cannot be regarded, philosophically at least, as the 'answer' to the conflicting theories of rights outlined above; the Convention could be regarded either as the legal expression of moral rights which already exist (assuming one agrees with the content of the rights set out within it) or as a brand-new set of legal rights, which those living in states signing up to the Convention are now entitled to enjoy. However, the fact that 45 countries, with significantly different religious and political histories, have signed it would suggest that, at the least, the Convention embodies notions widely held in Europe as to what is due to human beings by nature of their humanity.

Given that the UK signed the Convention back in 1951, those living within the jurisdiction of the UK have, in theory at least, benefited from the protections set out in the Convention for over 50 years. However, in practice, not many people are likely to go to the European Court of Human Rights in Strasbourg in order to challenge perceived breaches of the Convention – and until the year 2000 this was the only practical means of enforcing those rights. Moreover it is probably fair to say that few individuals, whether patients or health professionals, would have been able to recite the rights protected by the Convention. However, when the Human Rights Act 1998 came into force on 2 October 2000, all public authorities (including NHS bodies) were given the express statutory duty of respecting those Articles of the Convention cited in the 1998 Act and all individuals were given the right to take action in UK courts if those rights were not respected. The rights protected by the Convention thus assumed a far greater prominence than ever before.

The Articles of the Convention

The Articles of the Convention that are of most potential significance to those working in healthcare are set out in Table 4.1. Unsurprisingly, they are written in very general terms, and it is therefore necessary to look at the vast body of European Court case law which has built up over the past 50 years, together with English case law since October 2000, to see how these general propositions have been applied to healthcare.[5] However, while a close examination of the case law is crucial for reasons of interpretation, it would be a great mistake to think of the Convention as only being of relevance when patient–health professional relationships have collapsed to the extent that legal action is contemplated. While the Convention can certainly be used as a means of enforcing minimum standards through the courts, it also provides a valuable tool to enable health professionals to deal with ethical dilemmas, even (or indeed especially) where legal action is unlikely to be contemplated. The rest of this chapter will focus on this second use of the Convention, using the elucidation of the meaning of the Articles provided by the case law to demonstrate how those Articles can help in handling common primary care dilemmas. As will become clear, the Convention will rarely give 'yes/no' answers, unless by chance an identical issue has been considered by the courts in the recent past. What it will do is provide a framework to analyse the dilemma, particularly where competing rights are being asserted.

Table 4.1 Relevance of European Convention on Human Rights Articles to the NHS		
Article	*Rights protected by Article*	*Possible areas of relevance for NHS*
Article 2	The right to life, including a 'negative' prohibition on the intentional taking of life and a 'positive' obligation on states to take appropriate action to safeguard life	End-of-life decisions; suicide prevention; referral and resource allocation decisions
Article 3	The right to freedom from inhuman and degrading treatment	Very poor quality care; treatment without consent
Article 5	The right to liberty	Detention under the Mental Health Act 1983
Article 6	The right to have one's civil rights and obligations determined by a court	Professional disciplinary hearings where the right to practise is in jeopardy
Article 8	The right to respect for one's private and family life. This includes both 'negative obligations' not to interfere with an individual's privacy or family life and 'positive obligations' to take appropriate action to promote respect for these areas. 'Private life' has been very widely defined to include an individual's 'physical and psychological integrity'.	Confidentiality; access to treatment; appropriate involvement of families in a patient's care. Probably the most important Article for the NHS
Article 12	The right to marry and found a family	Access to fertility services
Article 14	The right to freedom from discrimination in the enjoyment of other Convention rights	Access to services where this is limited by potentially discriminatory criteria such as age

Confidentiality and information-sharing

A classic 'rights' dilemma in all parts of the NHS is posed by the issue of confidentiality and data-sharing. While both the common law of England and codes of professional ethics emphasise the importance of maintaining patient confidentiality, both recognise that there may be exceptional circumstances where confidential information may legitimately be shared without the consent, or even against the will, of the patient, for example, where information known only to a GP or health visitor might, if disclosed to social services or the police, protect others from serious harm. How can such dilemmas be analysed in terms of the European Convention?

The key here, as in many healthcare cases, is Article 8: the right to respect for one's private and family life. Article 8 is known as a 'qualified right': while Article 8(1) sets out an individual's *prima facie* right to respect in these areas, Article 8(2) sets out the (strictly circumscribed) circumstances in which those rights may legitimately be curtailed by the state. In order for any interference with Article 8(1) rights to be permissible, three criteria must be met.

- The interference must be in accordance with the domestic (i.e. English) law. Thus any action that would breach the common law of confidentiality, for example, could not be justified under Article 8(2).
- The interference must have a legitimate aim, and the aims that are acceptable are specified in the Article. Those of most relevance in healthcare cases include the aim of protecting the rights and freedoms of others and the aim of protecting health.
- Finally, and crucially, the interference must be 'necessary in a democratic society'. This terminology has been interpreted in the courts essentially as meaning 'the action is proportionate'. One way of dealing with this is to ask oneself whether the same legitimate aim could be met in a way which intrudes less on the individual's right to respect for their private and family life. If there *is* an alternative, less intrusive, method of achieving that aim, then the method which impacts more on the individual's Article 8(1) rights is unlikely to be proportionate.

An example of how the European Court of Human Rights has applied this three-part test to breaches of confidentiality that allegedly infringe Article 8 rights is found in the case of *MS v Sweden*.

MS v Sweden

ECHR Application 20837/92, 27/08/1997

MS's medical records had been disclosed by a clinic, without her knowledge, to the social security authorities to assist in determining her claim to compensation for a workplace injury. The Court held that the disclosure of medical records for a different purpose from that for which they were compiled, without the patient's consent, did constitute an interference with her Article 8(1) rights. However, this interference was justified under Article 8(2) in that it was (1) in accordance with Swedish law and was a foreseeable consequence of MS's compensation claim; (2) was in accordance with a legitimate aim (the economic wellbeing of the country); and (3) was necessary in a democratic society, because the effective safeguards against abuse in Swedish law meant that the communication of the records for a legitimate aim was not a disproportionate measure.

More generally, however, the Court emphasised the importance to be placed on clinical confidentiality, suggesting that close scrutiny will be given to whether disclosure in any particular case is proportionate.

> The Court reiterates that the protection of personal data, particularly medical data, is of fundamental importance to a person's enjoyment of his or her right to respect for private and family life as guaranteed by Article 8 of the Convention. Respecting the confidentiality of health data is a vital principle in the legal systems of all the Contracting Parties to the Convention. It is crucial not only to respect the sense of privacy of a patient but also to preserve his or her confidence in the medical profession and in the health services in general. The domestic law must afford appropriate safeguards to prevent any such communication or disclosure of personal health data as may be inconsistent with the guarantees in Article 8 of the Convention.

In many cases, there may be little doubt as to the lawfulness and legitimate aim of the proposed interference with an individual's Article 8 rights and the key issue will therefore be whether the proposed action is proportionate. In 2002, in the case of *R (on the application of S) v City of Plymouth,* the English Court of Appeal summarised all the competing rights involved where a mother wanted access to the medical and social care records of her incapacitated adult son in order to fulfil her role effectively as his nearest relative under the Mental Health Act 1983.[6] These included the:

- Article 8 rights of the son on both sides of the equation (his right to have his privacy respected, together with his right to respect for his family life, exemplified through the appropriate involvement of his mother with his care)
- Article 8 rights of the mother to be involved in her son's care
- Article 6 rights of the mother to have the information she needed if her right to act as her son's nearest relative were to be challenged in court, as social services proposed.

The Court then effectively drew up a shopping list of relevant factors to weigh in the balance when considering these conflicting rights and hence in determining whether disclosure would be 'proportionate'.

> These are the confidentiality of the information sought; the proper administration of justice; the mother's right of access to legal advice to enable her to decide whether or not to exercise a right which is likely to lead to legal proceedings against her if she does so; the rights of both C [the son] and his mother to respect for their family life and adequate involvement in decision-making processes about it; C's right to respect for his private life; and the protection of C's health and welfare. In some cases there might also be an interest in the protection of other people, but that has not been seriously suggested here.

In this case, a majority of the Court of Appeal held that the balancing exercise should lead to the disclosure to the mother of the information already accorded to her legal and medical advisors. Lady Justice Hale, who gave the leading judgment, noted in particular that 'there is a clear distinction between disclosure to the media with a view to publication to all and sundry and disclosure in confidence to those with a proper interest in having the information in question'. While both the remaining Court of Appeal judges agreed with Lady Justice Hale's analysis of the legal issues involved, one judge, however, held that the balance should be struck differently, with disclosure permitted only to the expert advisors and not to the mother.

This case demonstrates that in cases of competing rights there will rarely be one obvious answer: although all three Court of Appeal judges agreed on the form of balancing exercise to be undertaken and that some form of disclosure of the confidential information would be proportionate, there was disagreement as to the extent of that disclosure.

Nevertheless, the Convention does provide a framework to ensure all competing rights are properly considered and balanced, even if inevitably those performing the subsequent balancing act may not always come to the same conclusion.

Right to treatment and resource allocation

A second common area of concern in primary care is the question of how to balance potentially infinite and competing needs for care in a background of finite resources. This dilemma will arise both for those involved in commissioning services for all local residents and in individual decisions as to whether to refer a particular patient to secondary care.

Before the Human Rights Act 1998 came into force, there was much academic discussion as to whether an absolute right to treatment could be deduced from the Convention, either in terms of a right to life-saving treatment under Article 2 or more widely in terms of a right to any kind of treatment under Article 8. The European Court had already made clear that states have a positive obligation under Article 8 to *promote* respect for an individual's private life (as well as refraining from interfering with it) and that private life includes the concept of 'physical and psychological integrity'.[7] It therefore seemed at least theoretically possible that Article 8 could be used to argue that the state had a positive duty to take action, which would enhance an individual's physical and psychological integrity – a duty that would encompass virtually all health and social care.

Doubt as to the likelihood of Article 2 being used successfully to argue for the right to life-saving treatment, however expensive or unorthodox, has been cast by the European case of *Scialacqua v Italy*.[8] The European Commission of Human Rights (which until 1998 acted as an initial filter for claims made to the European Court) rejected a claim that the Italian authorities had breached Article 2 by refusing to refund the cost of allegedly life-saving herbal medicines because they were not included on the list of officially recognised medicines. While reserving judgment as to whether Article 2 could, in any case, be held to require states to provide particular treatments that were essential in order to save lives, the Commission commented that 'the provision cannot be interpreted as requiring States to provide financial cover for medicines which are not listed as officially recognised medicines'. Although the judgment did not explicitly refer to the issue of resources, the Commission's endorsement of the Italian system of an 'official list' of available drugs implicitly accepted the legitimacy of the need for states to control healthcare resources. Earlier cases on the scope of the positive obligation to take action to safeguard life under Article 2 have also made clear that the nature of this obligation cannot be absolute, but must have regard to whether the action being demanded would pose a disproportionate burden on the public authority concerned.[9]

The arguments in relation to Article 8 have, more recently, been definitively rejected in the English courts in the much publicised case of Yvonne Watts,[10] who sought reimbursement of the cost of a hip replacement operation, which she had undergone in France in order to bypass English waiting lists. The High Court judge held that even if Article 8 was relevant when considering access to treatment, any positive duty to promote the individual's mental or physical wellbeing was subject to the need to strike a fair balance between the needs of the individual and the needs of society. Thus any right to treatment 'would be qualified by the authority's right to determine healthcare priorities in the light of its limited resources'. He further rejected out-of-hand the claim that the pain suffered by Mrs Watts while waiting for her operation could constitute inhuman or degrading treatment, as prohibited by Article 3 of the Convention.

This decision demonstrates the pragmatism of the English courts, which are unlikely to seek to impose duties on the NHS that in practice would be impossible to meet. However, the fact that no absolute right to treatment can be deduced from Article 8 does not mean that the Article is irrelevant in making resource allocation or referral decisions. There have been a number of cases where the courts have taken into account *how* an authority has come to the decision under challenge and in particular whether it has taken proper account of individuals' Convention rights as part of that process.[11] Thus, while neither Article 2 nor Article 8 will *compel* authorities to provide treatment in all cases, they do require that the duty to take reasonable action to safeguard life and to promote patients' physical and psychological integrity is always considered seriously when coming to difficult decisions about competing priorities.

Article 14, which prohibits discrimination in the enjoyment of Convention rights and hence requires that all individuals are treated equally in areas covered by the Convention, is also potentially very relevant. If treatment is likely to promote a patient's physical and psychological integrity (and hence comes within the *scope* of Article 8, even if the needs of the community 'trump' the needs of the individual in this particular case), then Article 14 requires that the criteria used to determine access to that treatment are non-discriminatory. If, for example, a certain treatment were to be made available only to patients below a certain age or only to patients living in a certain area, then the onus would be on the health professionals involved in making that decision to demonstrate that there was a justifiable explanation for such distinctions. Thus age limits where the clinical evidence is clear that effectiveness of the treatment falls dramatically with age would probably be acceptable (although it might be necessary to demonstrate that any case would be looked at on its own merits), while an arbitrary age limit, imposed only to conserve resources, would almost certainly be in breach of the Convention.

Finally, Articles 2, 3 and 8 of the Convention, while not giving absolute rights to treatment, may well be relevant in determining the *form* that care and treatment takes as shown in the case of two disabled young women.

R (on the application of (1) A, (2) B (by their litigation friend the Official Solicitor), (3) X, (4) Y) v East Sussex County Council & the Disability Rights Commission (interested party) [2003] EWHC 167 Admin, 18/02/2003

The High Court was asked to determine the issue of whether two very disabled young women had a right under the ECHR to be lifted manually by their carers, rather than with the use of a hoist. The judge held that in such cases the Convention rights of both the disabled individuals and of their carers must be considered, with the rights of neither side automatically 'trumping' the others.

Where a failure to lift manually might threaten the women's absolute rights under Article 2 or Article 3 (for example, in the case of a fire or where they might otherwise be left in an undignified or distressing situation for an unacceptably long period of time), manual lifting would be required regardless of the impact on the carers. In other cases, however, where both parties' Article 8 rights were engaged, a balancing exercise would have to be undertaken where the rights of all concerned to respect for their personal and psychological integrity (as exemplified by the women's need to have their human dignity maintained and the carers' rights not to suffer avoidable injury) should be taken into account. The fact that the carers were being paid to provide a professional service was neither here nor there: a fair balance between the competing interests must be struck. Factors to be taken into account when striking this balance included: the possible methods of avoiding or minimising the risk of harm to the carer; the context of the particular lift, such as its frequency; the likelihood and severity of the risk to the carer; and the impact on the disabled person.

Disputes between health professionals and patients' families

A third common dilemma in primary care, as in secondary care, is found when there is a lack of agreement between health professionals and parents as to the most appropriate care for a child. In Convention terms, this can be analysed as a conflict between the child's Article 8 rights to respect for his or her physical or psychological integrity (in the form of the best possible care) and the Article 8 rights of both parent and child to have their family life respected (in leaving such decisions to the child's family). While the European Court has made emphatically clear that the rights of a child should always take precedence of those of the parent, this does not mean that the parent's rights are completely disregarded.[12] In particular, the parent has a very clear right to be properly involved in any decisions concerning their child's care, even if ultimately the decision is taken out of their hands, for example through a court declaration. The case of *Glass v UK*, which was heard in Strasbourg in 2004, made these points abundantly clear.

Glass v UK
ECHR Application 61827/00, 09/03/2004

David Glass, a very severely disabled teenager, had been admitted to hospital on a number of occasions throughout 1998. On the first occasion, the clinicians treating him believed that he was dying and that it was no longer appropriate to offer intensive care. His family were very unhappy with this advice and, in fact, David did recover and was able to go home, although he had to be re-admitted on a number of occasions. On one of these occasions, one of the doctors treating David recorded in his notes that his mother had agreed to the use of morphine to relieve David's distress and that court involvement to resolve the conflict over his treatment was therefore not necessary.

In October 1998, the doctors believed that David had now reached a terminal phase of his illness and that he should be given diamorphine for pain relief. This was done against the strongly expressed views of the family and a DNR notice was placed in David's notes without consulting his mother. The dispute between the family and the hospital resulted in physical violence against the doctors, with Mrs Glass intervening personally to resuscitate her son. Again, David in fact

---

Continued

recovered and was discharged home. Mrs Glass alleged that both her own Article 8 rights and those of her son had been breached.

The European Court agreed that David's Article 8 rights had been breached, holding as follows.

- The administration of diamorphine to a minor, against the wishes of his legal proxy, interfered with his Article 8(1) rights to respect for his private life, in particular his right to 'physical integrity'. Given this finding, the Court held that it was unnecessary to consider whether or not David's mother's right to respect for her family life was engaged.
- The question to be resolved was therefore whether that interference with David's Article 8(1) rights could be justified under Article 8(2). To be justified, such interference must be in accordance with the law, in pursuit of a legitimate aim and necessary in a democratic society.
- While the aim pursued by the doctors (that of David's best interests, as determined by their clinical judgment) was a legitimate one, the actions taken by the hospital were not necessary in a democratic society because they had failed to seek High Court authorisation of their decision to treat David with diamorphine against Mrs Glass's wishes. The doctors had already considered the possibility of seeking High Court involvement at an earlier stage: the fact that they did not in fact do so contributed to the situation in October. Moreover, the European Court was not convinced that the need to provide diamorphine in October constituted such an emergency that High Court involvement could not be sought at that stage.

The circumstances of the *Glass* case were clearly extreme. However, the wider implications that parents have a right to be fully and appropriately involved in their child's care, particularly where there are differing views as to what constitutes the child's best interests, will resonate in secondary care and primary care alike.

References

1 *See*, for example, chapters by Margaret MacDonald and HLA Hart in Waldron J, editor. *Theories of Rights*. Oxford: Oxford University Press; 1984.
2 Berlin I. Two concepts of liberty. In: Berlin I. *Four Essays on Liberty*. Oxford: Oxford University Press; 1979.

3 *See*, for example, Frankfurt H. Freedom of the will and the concept of a person. In: Watson G, ed. *Free Will* (Oxford Readings in Philosophy). Oxford: Oxford University Press; 1989. Also Dworkin G. *The Theory and Practice of Autonomy*. Cambridge: Cambridge University Press; 1988.

4 *See*, for example, Raz J. Rights-based moralities. In: Waldron J, ed. *Theories of Rights*. Oxford: Oxford University Press; 1984.

5 As the legal system in Scotland is distinct from that in England and Wales, the English case law cited here is not strictly binding in Scotland. However, since courts in both England/Wales and Scotland are bound by the Human Rights Act 1998 to take into account the case law of the European Court of Human Rights in Strasbourg, it is highly unlikely that a radically different approach would be taken in Scotland from that pursued in England and Wales.

6 *R (on the application of S) v City of Plymouth*. [2002] EWCA Civ 388, 26/03/2002.

7 *Botta v Italy*. ECHR Application 21439/93, 24/02/1998.

8 *Scialacqua v Italy*. ECHR Application 34151/96, 01/07/1999.

9 *Osman v UK*. ECHR Application 23452/94, 28/10/1998.

10 *R (on the application of Yvonne Watts) v (1) Bedford Primary Care Trust, (2) Secretary of State for Health*. [2003] EWHC 2228, 01/10/2003.

11 For example, *R (on the application of Haggerty) v St Helen's Council*. [2003] EWHC 803 Admin, 11/04/2003, where the Council was found to have acted in an exemplary fashion and *R (on the application of Goldsmith) v London Borough of Wandsworth*. [2004] EWCA Civ 1170, 27/08/2004, where decision makers were strongly criticised for failing to address their minds to Mrs Goldsmith's Article 8 rights.

12 *Yousef v The Netherlands*. ECHR Application 33711/96, 05/11/2002.

Chapter 5

Ethical considerations in the primary care of the elderly demented patient

Henk Parmentier, John Spicer and Ann King

> How am I today?
> Well, generally speaking,
> Standing up
> In a sitting down situation.[1]

Anon

Introduction

It has been said that of the four celebrated principles of medical ethics, respect for autonomy is pre-eminent.[2] If this is so, then nowhere is that respect potentially more challenged than in the care of persons who are to a greater or lesser degree restricted in their autonomous function. The literature on partial autonomy is rich and various, but a common theme runs through: that persons suffering from dementing processes are indeed restricted in their autonomy. Though we might attempt to follow Agich and Seedhouse in advancing the notion that autonomous choices should be maximally enhanced, to lack cognitive function is to affect the way in which the outside world is dealt with and free choice is made.[3, 4] That simple fact has a number of consequences, *inter alia:*

- proxies, whether relatives, professionals or advocates, may take decisions for such persons; and that could include decisions at the end of life, as well as the more mundane
- philosophical questions as to the nature of personhood and personal identity, or how we define ourselves as persons should be considered
- a question of how information pertaining to dementing patients, as with other incapacitous patients, should be handled.

This chapter will set these issues in the context of the primary care team charged with a responsibility for community care of the demented patient.

Case studies

We start by describing three case studies. They represent a spread of clinical and ethical content with which to guide further discussion on the subject.

Mrs A

Mrs A is a 94-year-old lady who lives in a care home. She was diagnosed with dementia of the Alzheimer's type 15 years ago. At present she is severely demented and unable to communicate. Physically she is in a frail condition and needs full nursing care and help with feeding. Her son is her only relative.

Before she was diagnosed with dementia, Mrs A was a strict vegan. However, in the first few years after the diagnosis of dementia was made, she lived by herself and was known to eat meat, and she continued to do so.

Recently she was visited by a member of Vegan Society, who was shocked to see that she was not on a strict vegan diet. He insisted to the medical team that her diet should change. The medical team was reluctant to change it due to her frail physical status. Her son expressed no opinion.

Mr B

Mr B is a 67-year-old man. He was diagnosed with cerebro-vascular dementia several years ago. He is unable to speak. He is in need of full nursing care. In the past, he has expressed the wish to his relatives that he did not want any 'heroic treatments'.

Now, due to increased risk of aspiration, a visiting consultant suggests inserting a PEG (percutaneous endoscopic gastrostomy) tube so Mr B can start on liquid food infused via the tube.

Mrs C

Mrs C is an 82-year-old lady. She was diagnosed with moderate dementia. She lives at home with her 86-year-old husband. He is providing 24-hour care with the help of carers and district nurses.

Continued

> Due to a fall Mrs C seems to be in a lot of pain with her right hip. Without an X-ray of her hip it will be difficult to exclude a hip fracture.
>
> Both the patient and the husband are adamant that she should not be admitted to hospital.

The scope and role of primary care for elderly demented patients

In the UK, the primary care of these sorts of patients takes place in two different types of environment. Many patients with dementia are cared for at home, principally by carers who are also relatives, but also by extended primary care teams including GPs, community nurses, social care staff, physiotherapists, speech and language therapists, and many others. Such teams need to work well together to offer the best care to individual patients.[5] Other demented patients live in residential facilities, which may have a primarily mentally or physically frail clientele. The skills of the same types of professionals are brought together to provide primary care, depending on the needs of the individual residents. This rather basic distinction between living in one's home and living in an institution has enormous ethical impact, which will be discussed further below.

At the beginning of the 21st century in the UK, few demented patients reside in hospitals or other secondary care institutions. That said, advice for these patients is also usually available from specialist physicians, nurses and psychiatrists.

Teamwork involving various professionals seems to be a key aspect of care of the elderly mentally frail patient for one reason above most others. Haggerty *et al* summarise the interprofessional aspects of continuity of care to patients and their families as follows: that the providers of care should know what has happened before agreeing between them on plans of management, and that providers who know the patient should care for them in the future.[6]

The great claim of primary care in the UK is continuity of care and sustained patient–professional relationships over time. In the care of the demented patient, such an ideal appears to be of value as knowledge of the 'pre-morbid' patient and his or her wishes, values and choices reinforces the notion of continuing personal identity.

In practical terms, such continuity has been under some recent threat. Social care provision is variable in breadth and depth around the UK, or even within different districts. To some extent, population mobility and flux has eroded the traditional long-term relationship between GP and patient. More specifically, for example, changes to GP out-of-hours provision may mean that the visiting practitioner has no previous knowledge of the patient. In addition, information services such as NHS Direct are clearly of little value to the patient who has limited cognitive abilities.

Primary care teams[7] who care for demented patients also need to consider issues around the end of life, providing holistic care, formal treatment options and many other issues that have an ethical substructure.

An initial ethical overview

Let us return to the three cases outlined earlier and first consider a rather basic philosophical question, which might appear startling – Is Mrs A a person?

The answer to the question seems almost self-evident. She is a person because she is alive, it might be argued! Much attention has been given to the issue of when a 'personhood' might begin, as a result of consideration of abortion, interrupted conception and other allied activities, and for the moment those issues will be left aside.[8] But a related discussion should be engendered as to if and when personhood might change, or even end, in the context of a patient who is demonstrably alive, for to do so is to examine the conceptual foundations of autonomy.

Descriptions of cases have been documented over many centuries and useful summaries have been given by Harris[9] and Evans.[10] One of the difficulties for clinicians in reviewing this kind of literature is synthesising the pure reason of philosophy with clinical experience, a task admirably sought and delivered by Hughes.[11] His analysis of the demented patient seems admirable and here we seek to amplify it in the context of primary care.

A demented patient may not, as Locke would have it, be considered to be 'a thinking intelligent being, that has reason and reflection, and can consider itself as itself, the same thinking thing in different times and places'.[12] If nothing else, these qualities reflect a higher order of cognitive function, the very qualities degraded as the dementing process proceeds. At some point they may be there, but at another they can be said to be reduced and even non-existent. Parfit[13] takes this analysis a stage further and describes personal identity as being contingent on psychological continuities or connectedness. Such impaired continuities are the very problems often identified by the relatives of demented patients – when language such as 'he isn't the person he was' is used, there is a strong sense of the loss of psychological continuity.

Drawing on several other philosophers, Hughes constructs another, 'situated embodied agent', view of the demented patient. 'Situated' in this sense refers to a self placed in a family, culture and historical context. One can only view a person in the context of their personal narrative, which is defined by these factors – a person as part of a situation.

We are quite clearly embodied even if psychological continuities become fractured as a result of disease, and our bodies remain the link between our minds and the outside world: we are the product of both acting together.

'Agency' is a common term in the language of ethics generally to describe the person acting in a moral manner as distinction from, for example, animals or plants, which have no capacity for moral agency.[14] Whilst this function may be impaired, at least in advanced dementia, it is not absent and may fluctuate with time and treatment.[15]

So, Hughes is advancing a notion of dementia where personhood is maintained despite reduced cognitive function, which seems more in keeping with a primary care perspective, and which is ascribable to Mrs A and our other patients. The model of primary care is one in which the patient is seen and cared for in their own environment, at home, with relatives and friends; the care professionals will have cared for the patient's body and mind over many years even before the onset of dementia. Inevitably, there may come a time when the patient needs to be admitted to intermediate care facilities, as has occurred with Mrs A and Mr B, but in the UK these care homes remain within primary care. That decision will be considered more fully below, hinging as it does on a framework of autonomy.

Connectedness

The American Geriatrics Society has stated firmly that views expressed by patients prior to the onset of incapacitating illnesses should be respected.[16] This is particularly relevant in the context of end-of-life decisions, such as that faced by Mr B and his relatives. On the face of it, Mr B has declared in advance that 'heroic treatments' are not something he wishes to endure, having thought about it when capacitous. To respect that wish is to do several things.

- It is to accept tacitly a distinction between an 'extraordinary' treatment like a PEG and an 'ordinary' treatment, something rather less invasive or burdensome.
- It is also to acknowledge the patient's autonomy when making judgments about his best interests, recognising that these may not be based solely on his best medical interests. Although the visiting consultant

may advise the insertion of a PEG in the best medical interest of Mr B, this is inconsistent with his past expressed views. Presumably his relatives will bear witness to this by reporting it to the care staff and even by stating their opposition to the form of care planned.

- By respecting the choice of Mr B, his family and professional carers are respecting his life choices, goals and personal context. It is representative of the 'connectedness' of his life, despite the illness that ostensibly undermines it. In Parfit's terms, both Mrs A and Mr B have lost psychological continuity between their past and present lives – this is part of dementia. (By extension, it has been argued that prisoners who become demented while serving a sentence should not thereafter be freed.[17] Their connectedness with their crimes is still there.)

In a sense, this respect for choices is analogous to respect for the intentions of the dead. Under the law, intentions such as the disposal of property by means of a will are respected and executed, in a situation where the deceased can have no possible way of influencing the outcome.

Are there any arguments against the line taken above? Should Mr B be subjected to a PEG even against his previous wishes? Those who espouse the principle of sanctity of life – to preserve life at all costs – might raise just that question. Although there are variations on the principle, it requires the professionals to preserve Mr B's life by most means, whatever he might have said in advance. A professional decision to act in Mr B's best medical interests is consistent with this principle and elides the differences between ordinary and extraordinary treatments and interventions. Connectedness with his past intentions and continuity of thought would be ignored in such an action.

In any event, Mr B has made an advance statement, which few patients currently do before they become incapacitous. There is a potential complication for the primary care team, noted by Gallagher and Clark, which should be borne in mind if a more general move to writing advance statements comes about. Where patients like Mr B declare that certain intensive treatments are not their choice, that will inevitably mean that more patients will remain at home in their final illnesses. That may mean that primary care teams will be faced with more complex palliative care situations to deal with, challenging them to rise to the task of looking after patients who do not wish for secondary transfer.[18] That situation could give much scope for dissent within primary care teams: it could be argued that those in closest contact with the patient may be in the best position to represent his or her best interests to those who make clinical decisions, and that is fertile ground for conflict. (*See* Chapter 7 for a further discussion of this issue.)

Mrs A's situation is less dramatic but similar. The question arises again as to how much respect a previously held view should be accorded, although there is a subtle difference. It seems that in the early course of her illness, she changed her long-held view about veganism – an important principle to those who hold it and a personal ethical position that demands respect. Is it the case that the dementia from which Mrs A suffers has degraded her principles and her life view? In that case, should her care team respect her previous view and insist on maintaining her principles after diagnosis? In Lockean terms, she has lost her capacity for reason and reflection and, over time, can no longer make decisions. Being a vegan prior to the onset of dementia and being a vegan afterwards are two totally different states of affairs. By extension, the care team should feel no obligation to cooperate with the Vegan Society visitor.

It is possible, as Wicclair describes,[19] for a patient-centred care team to respect the particular preferences, values and interests of the patient and link such a respect to more modern clinical notions of care including partnership, shared endeavour and therapeutic alliance. The difficulty in applying such a view to Mrs A is in deciding when her personal preferences may be less valued because of her failing cerebral function or, more realistically, for the choices about her veganism to evolve as her illness evolves.

The notion of value is examined in more detail by Dworkin, who advances an analysis of 'critical interests' – interests that confer value on a person's life. That Mrs A can have little critical sense of the 'projects and plans' is almost a given in her mental state. However, based on this, her carers should not necessarily withdraw other aspects of her care from which she might derive benefit or even enjoyment (Dworkin memorably gives 'peanut and jelly sandwiches, basking in the sun, and recognising no-one' as examples).[20]

The stance of Mrs A's visitor merits some examination: his view is moral, in the sense of being a disapprobation of her care, although in reality such disapprobation can only be relevant if undertaken by the moral agent herself.[21] In the absence of her own overtly autonomous decision, his insistence on a vegan diet cannot be judged to be in her best interests since they are clearly independent of her diet. In any event, it might be questioned just how much the content of her diet should be open for discussion beyond members of the care team.

Sharing information

The limits of information sharing are often discussed with respect to capacitous patients, but Hughes and Louw draw professionals' attention to an aspect of dementia care not often addressed, that of confidentiality.[22] Even a cursory glance at the three case studies will illustrate that information about patients A, B and C is easily and routinely shared between care staff, and even more widely. For care staff, it is tempting to rationalise this behaviour as being obviously necessary in the best interests of the patient – after all, how can the professionals possibly look after the patient's complex needs without being aware of all aspects of their situation?

From first principles, a respect for confidentiality flows from a respect for autonomy; and autonomy can be usefully considered as dependent on adequate information, freedom from coercion and capacity. It could be argued that if our three patients lack capacity, then they cannot make autonomous decisions, and therefore are not entitled to confidential relationships with their healthcare professionals. That is a fairly logical line of argument but vulnerable to several flaws. Professional duty dictates that information about A, B and C should stay within the care team. It would be poor professional behaviour if such information should leak into the wider domain and such behaviour might be judged similar to the covert administration of drugs to incapacitous patients, as reported by Wong et al.[23]

However, in our case studies, a wide dissemination of confidential information about the people is not at issue; it is the relatively restricted dissemination of information among staff and/or relatives that warrants attention. A practical, or pragmatic, justification of this, based on best clinical interests, can be argued but lacks a certain theorisation.

Another justification for sharing information within the team lies in the relationship between the patients and their care professionals. Traditionally, the duty of confidence between the clinician and patient was conceived in person-to-person relationships. However, that does not recognise the nature of modern primary care, which is delivered by a team of professionals working together. It is more realistic to define the confidential relationship between the team and the patient. Furthermore, there is no qualitative difference between a team caring for a capacitous patient and one caring for an incapacitous patient.

Hughes and Louw argue from a different perspective that professional duties on information sharing, as exemplified by the General Medical Council (GMC) rules,[24] do not recognise patients as being embedded in social and professional relationships. The incapacitous patient is embedded in a unique way, by virtue of their condition, and thus confidentiality is not an overriding principle: it is best regarded as an index of trust.[25]

Both these lines of argument can plausibly be regarded as legitimising information sharing in the care of incapacitous patients.

Caring for Mrs C

The crisis Mrs C finds herself in will be immediately recognisable to any community healthcare professional. We see ethical issues surfacing that have been considered already. How do we define her best interests? Is she capacitous enough to refuse a necessary intervention? How influential is Mr C in his wife's decision-making? How does her decision match her previous, and present, life view? In practical terms, how will Mr C, or indeed the primary care team, cope with her care if she is maintained at home?

As ever, there are pragmatic approaches that may be of value. Mrs C's capacity must be assessed[26] and, if present, her decision respected whatever the consequences. Her husband and the care team must find a way to offer care in these circumstances even if the outcome is poor. Clinicians can find this aspect particularly hard.

If she is not capacitous, Mrs C may yet have the decision-making ability to choose a surrogate,[27] in this case Mr C. Substituted judgment is not yet legally valid in England and Wales, but it is in other jurisdictions. If Mr C takes the decision that his wife should not be admitted to hospital on her behalf, it may not be in her best clinical interests and thus rather dubious morally. She is a vulnerable person over whom Mr C has a certain power as carer.[28] Among other things he may have an interpretive as well as a decisional role.

Care giving, a term usually applied to persons providing direct full-time social care, as opposed to 'clinical' professionals, is in many ways the foundation of support to elderly demented people. Care ethics as a field has sprung up in recent years, from feminist ethical roots,[29] to consider the relationship between caring as a personal or professional endeavour and moral theory. Care ethics is more concerned, as Verkerk memorably describes it, with 'the dangers of abandonment than interference' even though its roots have been challenged.[30]

Autonomy, traditionally interpreted, may be described as a rather absolutist notion. We have already said that if Mrs C is capacitous, her decision-making should be respected at all costs. But in fact such a construction sees her decisions as rather insular and insulated, and that is perhaps just not how things are generally. Mrs C, and the rest of humanity, makes her healthcare decisions in the context of her relationships. She cannot decide whether she is admitted to hospital without the knowledge, influence or even coercion of Mr C, and other family members. Put differently, her decisions are interdependent on her relationships with others.

So, if she is incapacitous, it is not a great leap to consider her family and carers involved in her decision, almost nested within it. At first sight, this is a different interpretation of respect for the principle of autonomy: one which is of particular relevance to caring relationships. Verkerk[31] terms this a 'relational autonomy,' not to simply invoke the relatives of patients, but more to indicate that autonomous decisions are related to others in the sense already described.

Clearly Mr C has a measure of understanding of his wife and thus any decisions she makes are partially referential to him. Furthermore, if her autonomy, as traditionally interpreted, is limited by her mental state, then that referencing takes a larger role. Her autonomous decisions are in some way shared with him. To a lesser extent, such shared decisions may happen with the primary care team members, or at least those with whom Mrs C has had a prior relationship of some sort. What emerges from this kind of discussion is a new interpretation of the traditionally absolutist notion of autonomy, which seems useful in the context of limited decisional capacity and particularly as applied to primary care.

The issue of whether Mrs C should be at home or in hospital has already been mentioned: it is fundamental, not merely as part of the decision about where she should be cared for, although that latter aspect might be said to exercise healthcare professionals to the greatest extent. Quite obviously, our decisions about where we should be spatially at any time are key autonomous decisions. A move, permanently or otherwise, from home to elsewhere has enormous personal ramifications. For Mrs C, it seems that move is unacceptable even in pursuit of her best medical interests.

However the wider issue of where the elderly mentally frail in general should be cared for exercises policy makers and health professionals alike, and it is an area of ethical interest. While it is clear that such patients should be cared for in facilities best suited to them, it might be asked whether the transfer to such facilities is always entirely without coercion or whether the preservation of care at home is restricted by resource or managerial reasons. Moreover, the practical effect in the case of Mrs C might be to leave her at home with a possible hip fracture, a state of affairs from which most clinicians will intuitively recoil, if only on the grounds of defensibility.

Adopting the tentative 'relational' autonomy approach allows Mrs C, her husband and the primary care team to blend views on her best interests and her decision-making to formulate an ethically robust placement, the nature of which will inevitably differ with individual circumstances. The situation will also change with the passage of time. It is generally accepted that autonomous decisions should be dynamic: that is to say able to change with changing circumstances. And thus even a 'shared' autonomous decision should he considered similarly. Watts *et al*[32] analyse this sort of issue from the point of view of risk, emphasising that these are fluid and complex situations – they evolve over time and demand healthcare interventions that are creative and respectful of the patient and their carers. The dynamic nature of autonomous decision-making is mirrored by the dynamic nature of an evolving, rather complicated family situation. On occasions, and not always obviously, there may be risk to other people as a result of the deteriorating mental state of the patient (for example, where memory loss leads to danger in the use of gas appliances). A consequentialist justification for transfer to a supervised facility is sometimes not hard to argue.

Conclusions

In this chapter, we have rehearsed some of the ethical issues surrounding the care of the elderly patient in primary care, with particular reference to the demented patient. Clear answers to the dilemmas described in the three case studies have purposefully not been offered, in favour of a more descriptive approach. Arguably, another route into analysis of these issues is empirical. What actually happens and is there a useful ethics that can be derived? Can ethics lead to codes of practice that are more realistically, and therefore we would argue, ethically informed?

We end this chapter by following the lead of three Swedish authors, who have worked empirically, and by supporting the view that it is the ethical discussion in the care team that is of the highest importance.[33] They offer a reflective tool as a means of achieving that aim: while the details of the framework are not crucial, and many others are known and found more or less useful, the nature of the discussion that takes place leads to an ethical competence and even an ethical creativity in defining the care of this most challenging population.

From this rather discursive aim, we return to the representations of autonomy that have been discussed. We started with the well-known descriptor of the principle of autonomy as being predominant and absolute, and have ended with a differing interpretation: one more acknowledging of the shared process and results. This interpretation is offered in particular reference to those in primary care who may have longer-term relationships with patients and have something to gain from an understanding of the ethics of care.

References

1 Extract from unpublished poem, collected by John Killick. *Dementia: mind, meaning and person* (Conference abstracts; 2002). Newcastle upon Tyne. Philosophy Special Interest Group of Faculty for the Psychiatry of Old Age, Royal College of Psychiatrists.
2 Beauchamp T, Childress D. *Principles of Biomedical Ethics*. 4th ed. Cambridge: Cambridge University Press; 1994.

3 Agich GJ. *Dependence and Autonomy in Old Age*. Cambridge: Cambridge University Press; 2003.

4 Seedhouse D. *Ethics: the heart of healthcare*. New York: John Wiley; 1998.

5 And may not always do so: *see* Chapter 4.

6 Haggerty JL, Reid RJ, Freeman GK, Starfield BH, Adair CE. Continuity of care: a multidisciplinary review. *BMJ*. 2003; **327**: 1219–21.

7 Whalley LJ. Dementia: the key issues for primary care. *The New Generalist*. 2004; **2**(Winter): 4 (a review of diagnosis and investigation only).

8 The reader is directed to Dunstan GR, Seller MJ, eds. *The Status of the Human Embryo: perspectives from moral tradition*. London and Oxford: King's Fund and Oxford University Press; 1988 or Glover J. *Causing Death and Saving Lives*. Harmondsworth: Penguin; 1994 for discussions of this area.

9 Harris J. *The Value of Life: an introduction to medical ethics*. London: Routledge; 1997. Chs 1, 10, 11.

10 Evans M. Some ideas of the person. In: Greaves D, Upton H, eds. *Philosophical Problems in Health Care*. Aldershot: Avebury Publishing; 1997. Ch. 2.

11 Hughes JC. Views of the person with dementia. *J Med Ethics*. 2001; **27**: 86–91.

12 Locke J (1689). *An Essay Concerning Human Understanding*. Nidditch PH, ed. Oxford: Oxford University Press; 1975. Also quoted in Chapter 3, Conceptions of persons and dementia. In: Greaves D. *The Healing Tradition: reviving the soul of Western medicine*. Oxford: Radcliffe Medical Press; 2004 (an excellent review of the issue).

13 Parfit R. *Reasons and Persons*. Oxford: Oxford University Press; 1986.

14 Animals as moral agents are not totally discounted: *see* Coetzee JM. *The Lives of Animals*. Princeton: Princeton University Press; 1999 and Singer P. All animals are equal. In: Singer P, Regan T, eds. *Animal Rights and Human Obligations*. 2nd ed. Englewood Cliffs: Prentice Hall; 1989.

15 Gauthier S. Drugs for Alzheimer's Disease and related dementias. *BMJ*. 2005; **330**: 858–9.

16 Lynn J. Measuring quality of care at the end of life: a statement of principles. *J Am Geriatrics Soc*. 1999; **45**: 526–7.

17 Fazel S, McMillan J, O'Donnell I. Dementia in prison: ethical and legal implications. *J Med Ethics*. 2002; **28**: 156–9.

18 Gallagher P, Clark K. The ethics of surgery in the elderly demented patient with bowel obstruction. *J Med Ethics*. 2002; **28**: 105–8.

19 Wicclair MR. Ethics, community and the elderly: healthcare decision-making for incompetent elderly patients. In: Parker M, ed. *Ethics and Community in the Healthcare Professions*. New York: Routledge; 1999.

20 Dworkin R. *Life's Dominion*. New York: Knopff; 1993.

21 Emmet D. *Rules, Roles and Relations*. Basingstoke: Macmillan; 1966.

22 Hughes JC and Louw SJ. Confidentiality and cognitive impairment: professional and philosophical ethics. *Age and Ageing*. 2002; **31**: 147–50.

23 Wong JG, Poon Y, Hui EC. 'I can put medicine in his soup, Doctor!' *J Med Ethics*. 2005; **31**(5): 2625.

24 General Medical Council. *Confidentiality: protecting and providing information*. London: GMC; 2000.

25 *See* Chapter 1 and also Smith C. Understanding trust and confidence: two paradigms and their significance for health and social care. *J App Phil*. 2005; **22**(3): 299–316.

26 A full description of the clinical assessment of legal capacity is beyond the scope of this chapter, but the reader is directed to the *BMA Guide to Assessment of Capacity* published jointly by the BMA and the Law Society as a useful source in 1999.

27 Brauner DJ, Cameron Muir J, Sachs GA. Treating non-dementia illnesses in patients with dementia. *JAMA*. 2000; **283**(24): 3230–5.

28 Norberg A. Ethics in the care of the elderly patient with dementia. In: Gillon R, ed. *Principles of Healthcare Ethics*. New York: John Wiley; 1994.

29 *See*, for example, Fry ST. The role of caring in nursing ethics. In: Holmes HB, Purdy LM, eds. *Feminist Perspectives in Medical Ethics*. Bloomington, IN: Indiana University Press; 1992.

30 Allmark P. Can there be an ethics of care? In: Fulford KWM, Dickenson DL, Murray TH. *Healthcare Ethics and Human Values*. Malden, MA: Blackwell; 2002.

31 Verkerk M. The care perspective and autonomy. *Med Healthcare & Phil*. 2001; **4**: 289–94.

32 Watts DT, Cassel CK, Howell T. Dangerous behaviour in a demented patient: preserving autonomy in a patient with diminished competence. In: Mappes TA and DeGrazia D. *Biomedical Ethics*. 4th ed. Boston: McGraw Hill; 1996.

33 Bolmsjo IA, Sandman L, Andersson E. Everyday ethics in the care of elderly people. *Nursing Ethics*. 2006; **13**(3): 259–63.

Chapter 6

Setting boundaries: a virtue approach to the clinician–patient relationship in general practice

Peter Toon

> The power of a man's virtue should not be measured by his special efforts but by his ordinary doing.
>
> Blaise Pascal

Introduction

At one time people thought medical ethics consisted of medical etiquette, for example, not criticising colleagues or working with unlicensed practitioners, taking the precautions needed to avoid falling foul of the General Medical Council (GMC), and not advertising, doing abortions or engaging in sexual liaisons with patients. In the 1970s, a more formal approach drifted across the Atlantic from the USA as 'bioethics'. There was (and to some extent still is) a naively rationalist view among medical educationalists that having the philosophical skills needed to analyse the rights and duties in a situation or to evaluate the consequences of a course of action will make doctors behave better. Some even believed that it was unnecessary to grapple with deontology and consequentialism – all you needed were the four principles of autonomy, justice, beneficence and non-maleficence,[1] and all would be well. Emphasis on the duties of beneficence and respect for autonomy has been institutionalised in the GMC's *Duties of a Doctor*.[2] These make depressing reading. They offer a list of demanding duties and only a passing reference to the unspecified rewards and privileges of being a doctor. One may well ask, 'Why does anyone bother to be a doctor?'

While this has been going on in medicine, in philosophy there has been a revival in virtue ethics. Ethics from Aristotle[3] until the Enlightenment largely focused on the study of the personal qualities required to act rightly. For Aquinas[4] these were 'the habits (or disposition) to act rightly according to reason'. In the last 200 years rationalism has led the focus to be on 'according to reason' rather than on habits or dispositions. But over the last 30 years or so various authors, most notably MacIntyre,[5] have returned to the study of virtue.

MacIntyre argues that virtues are cultivated in 'practices' – coherent and complex socially established cooperative human activities through which non-material 'internal goods' are realised through the pursuit of excellence. While external goods (money, possessions, power, prestige) are finite objects of competition, internal goods (knowledge, skill, excellence) are not diminished by being shared.

MacIntyre believes that virtues are cultivated through striving to achieve these goods through practices and the specific virtues required will be different in different practices. Another way of looking at this is that different 'moral roles' (parent, teacher, doctor, soldier) require and develop particular virtues – or at least a particular pattern of virtues.[6] Nussbaum and Sen[7] suggest that the virtues are characteristically the qualities needed to face the challenges of life successfully (and, of course, the challenges one faces depend in part on the roles one takes).

Virtue ethics is often contrasted with deontology, but Hursthouse[8] has suggested that while deontology is not a sound basis for ethics, we can nevertheless define certain 'v-rules' – principles which although not rigid like deontological rules, nevertheless can be used as 'rules of thumb' that indicate lines of action generally likely to lead to flourishing, such as telling the truth and respecting the property rights of others.

A key concept in virtue ethics is *phronesis* or 'practical wisdom' – for Aristotle the one virtue that was both moral and intellectual. It is the ability to perceive situations from a virtuous perspective and to analyse the virtuous course of action. It allows right action 'according to reason'; it includes but is not limited to the skills of ethical analysis cultivated in the traditional teaching of bioethics.

Medicine is, in MacIntyrean terms, a 'practice' – indeed it is one of the examples which he uses in his account of what a practice is. Virtue ethics emphasises the benefits to the agent, since virtuous actions are those that lead to flourishing and the good life. Many of the problems that have faced medicine cannot readily be solved by the application of externally imposed rules, but require that doctors have the personal qualities that we count as virtues. Virtue ethics therefore seems a promising approach to addressing the ethical problems of medical practice.

Applying virtue ethics

Medicine faces many ethical problems, but perhaps two of the most significant at present are:

- public concern about standards of practice and the orientation and values of practitioners
- poor morale among doctors, evidenced by problems in recruitment and retention as well as dissatisfaction among established practitioners.

The public concern was first voiced more than 20 years ago by writers such as Illich[9] and Kennedy,[10] although it has received new impetus in the last few years from the Bristol,[11] Alder Hey[12] and Shipman[13] cases. The fall in morale may in part be a consequence of this concern and deontological responses to it, which, by subjecting doctors to an increasingly demanding set of rules and procedures to monitor performance against those rules, many see as adding to already heavy burdens.

Perhaps virtue ethics offers a way out of this impasse.[14] In this chapter, I will begin to explore this possibility, focusing on one specific issue at the heart of general practice, dealing with patients 'who are or who believe themselves to be ill' (the British Medical Association's (BMA) General Practice Committee's definition of the core task of general practice). Anyone can bring any problem to their GP. Determining the boundaries of what the GP should do is therefore difficult and cannot be easily addressed by rules, since the cases are too varied. This is a problem where the virtue ethics approach is particularly relevant. I will therefore focus on this question: How does the virtuous GP act in situations at the boundaries of the role?

The rationale for the method

Like many issues in moral philosophy, proposals about the virtues include both claims of fact and claims of value. Suggestions that certain features constitute the good life, the life that is fully human (flourishing) are claims of value. The suggestion that certain qualities are needed to achieve such a life is a claim of fact. The two may be intertwined – courage may, for example, be needed both to achieve a good life and also to contribute to the good life in and of itself.

Answers to questions of fact, if they are to be generalisable, need to be based not on the reflection, philosophical analysis or observations of a single individual, but from data collected as widely and as representatively as possible. The meaning of flourishing as a medical practitioner is an issue of value to be addressed by philosophical reasoning, but defining the qualities needed for such flourishing is also at least partly empirical (only partly if having the qualities needed for flourishing is itself a constituent of flourishing), and so this too requires the collection of data.

Since, however, medicine is a cooperative human activity (a practice in the MacIntyrean sense), even its claims of value may be better elucidated by starting from the values expressed by those engaged in the practice and then subjecting these claims of value to critical philosophical analysis. I have therefore chosen to approach the problem by using methods that build on, but are not limited to, techniques used in qualitative empirical research.

The method

At a one-day research seminar,[15] I collected stories from a group of GPs (and one psychologist), which they felt illustrated some of the difficulties faced by GPs and the qualities needed to overcome them. I kept in touch with the group by e-mail and they gave me more stories and comments on these in this virtual dialogue. The stories are mostly not the classical 'ethical dilemmas' that you might find in textbooks on medical ethics, but practical, everyday problems. Because the clinician is unsure what to do they become stressed and an unwise action may harm the patient. Identifying 'v-rules' for these situations may therefore benefit both doctors and patients.

In this chapter, I will use some of these stories to explore the boundaries of what the virtuous GP should take on and also to test the more general hypothesis that virtue ethics, coupled with this type of qualitative research method, offers a useful way to develop primary care ethics.

The stories

Story 1: responding as a wise friend in authority

A young doctor, previously unknown to you, is discharged from hospital with her first baby, with severe anoxic brain damage. Her pharmacist husband is clearly distraught and cannot accept this event. You are asked to advise. You judge that this is going to destroy the parents' relationship and strongly advise the possibility of arranging adoption. It is accepted. (They then have two brilliant children and successful professional careers.)

The author defined the challenge posed by this story as: 'Have you the right to offer such a solution?' (it is interesting that the question is phrased deontologically, indicating the pervasiveness of this type of thinking in medicine).

Traditionally, the doctor's role is to cure or relieve illness, help patients avoid illness and help them understand and cope with their illness.[16] Doctors are granted certain powers by virtue of their professional role, for example, to prescribe medicines and to give permission for time off work. In this case, the doctor is not exercising any of these professional skills or socially granted powers. Providing advice in situations such as this lies outside the medical role, which is the cause for the anxiety underlying the question 'Have you the right to offer such a solution?' That the story was brought to a seminar several years after the incident suggests that, despite the favourable outcome, the doctor's advice given long ago caused continuing tension and uncertainty.

There may be medical facts about the prognosis of the child and other general facts about similar situations, for example, data on marital breakdown in families with mentally handicapped children, which fall within the doctor's professional expertise. The parents may rightly feel that a doctor will have seen other people in similar situations and that this makes his or her views particularly valuable. But it is nevertheless not a medical judgment. Rather the doctor is acting as anyone placed in a similar position might act, playing a role that a number of people might play – priests or ministers of religion, lawyers or social workers, a respected family friend or relative. The role is not specific to any profession – it is more akin to that of a wise friend than a professional.

Hypothesis 1: that the doctor acts as a wise friend

This story therefore suggests our first hypothesis that on some occasions, GPs are faced with situations that lie outside their professional role. In such situations they have to decide how to act as a 'wise friend'.

Doctors do become friends with their patients. This is particularly likely to happen to GPs who have relationships with individuals and families over many years and who live in the same community as their patients. Is the concept of friendship appropriate to this case?

Aristotle devotes two chapters of the *Ethics*[17] to a discussion of friendship and his work is an obvious place to look for ideas on this question. He points out what we would all agree with – that a principal characteristic of friendship is that the individuals involved take pleasure in each other's company. This does not seem to fit with our present case. Although there may be a particular affinity because the patient is a doctor and her husband a pharmacist, a profession closely allied to medicine, there is nothing to suggest that this type of friendship exists between the doctor and this family.

However, Aristotle also identifies friendships that exist between unequals. The examples he gives are of father and son, husband and wife (not one that would be seen as desirably unequal today!) and those in authority over their subordinates. None of these quite fit our example, but this nevertheless does seem to be a type of unequal friendship. If the doctor were faced with a similar challenge in his own personal life we would be surprised if he sought the opinion of a patient, unless a friendship of the commoner, equal type existed between them. Seeking advice from someone we would not presume to advise is a characteristic of unequal friendships.

Doctors are still seen by many as authority figures, albeit perhaps less than they were, and as having knowledge of issues of living that lie outside their professional training. To some extent this may be a psychodynamic projection, reflecting an understandable search for someone to lean on in trying circumstances (something that the patient here, even though a doctor herself, would by no means be immune to). But it is reasonable for a patient to think that doctors' professional lives (like those of the other professions mentioned above) give them experience of the challenges of living that help them to develop their practical wisdom. This may mean that their opinion is worth seeking in relation to problems of living that are not strictly medical.

Hypothesis 2: that this type of friendship is an unequal one

What are the qualities that the doctor needs to act virtuously in this type of unequal friendship with patients?

Some of these qualities follow logically from the discussion above. The advice offered by a wise friend must be wise advice. This implies sufficient knowledge of the world and of human behaviour to be able to make a sensible judgment on general grounds, which will include but go beyond formal, scientific evidence. It also implies the diligence to find out enough about the patient and the problems she faces to be able to apply this general knowledge to this particular situation.

In deciding whether to give advice and if so what advice to give, the wise friend must take account of whether he or she is qualified to give the advice. An important element in practical wisdom for the doctor faced with questions like these is self-knowledge. The doctor must be aware what they are doing. But applying this general knowledge to give advice on what course of action to take is not a matter of medical expertise but of human wisdom. The doctor has to be clear to themselves, when they are acting out of professional expertise and when they are acting in 'wise friend with authority' mode. Some of the disasters of previous decades – the incarceration of unmarried mothers in sub-normality hospitals in the UK, aversion therapy for homosexuals, the psychiatric treatment of dissidents in the USSR, among many others – have been in part a result of doctors failing to draw this distinction clearly. Not only was the decision in each case wrong, but it was made possible because doctors claimed expertise that they did not have.

Doctors have to make similar judgments when giving medical advice. Are they competent to do so? Knowing the limits to one's clinical competence is important, but so too is knowing the limits to one's practical wisdom outside of medicine. It is flattering to be asked to advise on a difficult question and doctors have to beware of responding to such flattery. This is an aspect of the virtue of humility, which does not mean a Heep-like self-deprecation, but a realistic assessment of one's faults and limitations.

The doctor also has to make a judgment about those seeking the advice and how they will respond to it. If, for example, the case is as suggested above, that they are looking for a father figure to take responsibility for a decision they prefer not to make themselves rather than a wise friend to give them counsel, then it may be unwise to give any advice. This may lead to recriminations. Anger is often projected in dependency relationships and looking for advice may be a disguised way of looking for someone to blame should things go wrong. Although patients do complain about medical advice and treatment (often for much the same reasons), this issue does not arise in the same way with strictly medical advice. Here roles and what constitutes reasonable practice are more clearly predefined.

Other insights flow from general ideas about the virtues of friends. The doctor must feel benevolent towards the patient, wishing them well and wanting the best for them, or a sound judgment cannot be made. Courage may sometimes be needed to voice a judgment on a difficult matter, particularly if the judgment is an unfashionable one. Going beyond the medical role can be risky.

Hypothesis 3: that a dispassionate assessment of one's own abilities and limitations, a realistic assessment of the patient's needs and aspirations, and sufficient knowledge of the world and the situation are elements of practical wisdom needed in this type of situation

Hypothesis 4: that benevolence and courage are important virtues in this situation

The account above could apply to any person facing such a dilemma in a professional or non-professional relationship. In what way (if any) does the fact that the 'wise friend' in this situation is a doctor influence the situation? By the nature of their work doctors are faced more often with people in difficult situations of this type and so responding to them may play a larger part in their lives than in those of other people.

Once such a situation arises, however, there is no alternative but to face it. To brush off the request for advice or to retreat into a formal medical role is not only an act of cowardice, but is itself a decision. To decide to do nothing is itself to do something. And the virtues required are similar whether the person asked for the advice is a doctor, a lawyer, a priest or a friend.

This points us to one way in which acting virtuously in this situation contributes to the flourishing of the doctor. To refuse to think about the matter is to limit one's potential for engaging with the realities of life and so to refuse to grow and develop as a person, surely one aspect of what it means to flourish. Clearly it is important that the doctor approaches the problem thoughtfully so as to be sure that the advice given is the best possible. By doing so not only does he or she do their best for the patient but also ensures that should their advice be followed and turn out to be wrong, he or she can at least console themselves with having done their best.

Hypothesis 5: that once faced with a request to act as a wise friend the doctor has no alternative to face up to it if he or she is to flourish

These hypotheses must be tested against other stories where the GP is faced with situations 'on the boundaries' to see whether they cover these too.

Story 2: responding as a good neighbour

> A doctor is called one evening to visit an elderly lady living alone and he finds that she is seriously ill with heart failure. Clearly she needs immediate admission to hospital, but she has no one to take care of her dog. Her neighbours are away and her only friends near by are allergic to dogs. He agrees to look after the dog overnight until a place can be found for it in kennels the next day.

This story caused a heated discussion. Was it appropriate for a doctor to take on such a responsibility?

It clearly lies outside the role of caring for 'those who are or who believe themselves to be ill', but the role of 'wise friend' defined in the last case does not seem appropriate here. Not much wisdom or authority (apart from a basic knowledge of the care of dogs and an ability to control them, which scarcely counts) are called for – even friendship does not seem particularly relevant. The role of undertaking a practical service for someone in trouble, of which this is an example, can perhaps be better thought of as that of the 'good neighbour' rather than wise friend in authority. Hypotheses 1 and 2 clearly do not therefore apply to this case, and we have a new hypothesis.

Hypothesis 6: that on some occasions GPs faced with situations that lie outside their professional role must decide whether and how to act as a 'good neighbour'

What are the virtues of a good neighbour? How does being a good neighbour contribute to the doctor's flourishing?

In our culture the archetype of the good neighbour is the Good Samaritan and in discussing the role one cannot ignore this figure and his virtues. The point of the story as recorded in the gospels is that the Samaritan responds to need on the basis of common humanity, rather than taking account of who the person is. He also shows a common-sense practicality – like the good paramedic, he administers first aid at the roadside and then gets the victim to a place where better care can be given. However, he also limits his involvement to what is practical – he does not abandon his business trip and other duties, but delegates care to the innkeeper, while ensuring that satisfactory care is provided by offering to foot the bill if necessary.

These virtues can be applied to good neighbourly acts performed by doctors.

Hypothesis 7: that the response of the good neighbour is not on the basis of a professional relationship but of common humanity

The virtuous response is immediate, practical and sensible but also limited to what is necessary – the good neighbour does not feel an obligation to take on responsibility for the whole world. This latter point is particularly important for doctors. The Good Samaritan probably only travelled occasionally from Jerusalem to Jericho and the probability of coming across victims of muggings was therefore not very high, even on that notoriously dangerous road. But doctors, by the nature of their work, come across an enormous quantity of human suffering and a large number of opportunities for acting as good neighbours. They would be swamped if they attempted to take on this burden. They have to make choices about when to act as a good neighbour and when to avert their gaze and walk on by. But these choices must also be made virtuously.

Like the Good Samaritan responding to human need, the virtuous doctor will decide which opportunities for good neighbourliness to respond to on the basis of need rather than favouring people of a particular race, religion or degree of personal charm. This requires the virtue of justice in a very similar way to that required to act virtuously in making rationing decisions, a rather different role of the doctor.

The nature and size of the task is important. Responses in the discussion were greatly (and reasonably) affected by whether or not the doctor (and/or his family) was a dog lover. Those that were not would have felt more inclined to be a good neighbour if the pet had been a canary! Other aspects of the doctor's situation are relevant too. If, for example, one of his children was terrified of dogs or his wife was allergic to dog hair, it would not have been virtuous to agree to look after the dog.

The temperate doctor will be temperate not just in avoiding excess alcohol, late nights and an overbooked diary which prevents him doing the job properly, but also in making temperate judgments about his own practical limitations. This is not just a question of practical wisdom, although that is important, but also involves right feelings – in doing what can be done with pleasure and enthusiasm, but also not feeling guilt about what cannot be taken on.

Responding to human need in this way can give the doctor, like other people, considerable satisfaction, as well as making the world a better place. It contributes both to individual and to corporate flourishing. But there must be limits. Motivations to enter medicine are varied, but a desire to make the world a better place is common – probably more common than is acknowledged. As a result doctors are at risk of seeking to take on too much responsibility, which can be a form of hubris, a refusal to acknowledge one's personal frailty and human limitations. Far from leading to flourishing, this can lead to a sense of resentment and burnout.

Hypothesis 8: that practical wisdom, benevolence, temperance and justice are important virtues in deciding what good neighbourly acts to take on

As well as the role being different, the virtues called upon to play it successfully are slightly different from those outlined in Hypothesis 5.

Although (because of the unity of the virtues) one can see how courage might be relevant to being a good neighbour, it does not seem so central; nor do temperance and justice appear so relevant to being a wise friend.

Story 3: responding as a wise friend to a request for good neighbourly action

Another story in which a health professional is faced with someone in need of a good neighbour illustrates how responding to a request for a good neighbour does not always involve doing everything yourself.

A psychologist is visiting a frail elderly couple to make an assessment. Rather surprisingly, at the end of the interview one of them asks, 'Can you cook chops?' Exploration of this rather strange question reveals that because they are unable to cook for themselves a carer usually comes in to get their meals. Today, however, the person who normally does their lunch is unavailable and no substitute has been provided, so they have no access to food until their carer comes to make supper. The response of the psychologist is to investigate the kitchen, which reveals that the fridge is almost empty – there are not even any chops for him to cook! He therefore makes the couple a cup of tea and some biscuits and rings the social services provider to complain about the neglect of them, doing so in the role of 'a psychologist from the health authority' (who ultimately pays the bill for the social services). A carer is on the doorstep with a full bag of shopping before he leaves!

In this case a request for a good neighbourly action is not responded to so much in the role of good neighbour (although the psychologist does produce tea and biscuits) as in the role of wise friend in authority, which in the long term is probably going to be of more benefit to the couple. If he had set to, gone shopping and made dinner himself, they would have had a good meal and he would have a warm glow of self-satisfaction, but the long-term situation would not have been improved. By addressing the underlying issue – poor organisation of cover for absent carers – he stood a chance of avoiding a recurrence of the problem.

Hypothesis 9: that practical wisdom is needed to decide what role – formal medical role, wise friend in authority or good neighbour – if any it is appropriate for a doctor to play in a given situation

Story 4: responding as a patron

An 18-year-old boy came to see me (brought along by his big brother) because he had recently breached a Community Service Order in relation to a burglary he committed the previous year and he was therefore facing a court appearance and likely imprisonment. I have known him, his brother and the rest of their family for 18 years and essentially they were asking if I would intervene with a request to the court to give him a last chance because of the rough times he has had in his life. These included the death of his mother when he was eight, his father's marriage to a step-mother with whom the boy has been in chronic conflict, and the recent death of his one surviving grandmother. He was by then estranged from his father and step-mother, and had in fact been living rough for a while (hence his breach of the Community Service Order), but had recently been taken in hand by his eldest brother who had volunteered to become *in loco parentis*.

The doctor who gave me this story commented that, 'Essentially, they were asking me to act not so much as a doctor but more like a good neighbour who just happened to know the family well enough to be able to affirm their story'.

In fact, with respect to the concepts discussed above, this seems not so much a matter of being a good neighbour, as in the case of the old lady with the dog, or as a wise friend in authority, for the doctor is being asked to intercede as a patron, a role that might have been very familiar to Aristotle and his colleagues in the ancient world and which has not yet disappeared even from our egalitarian society.

The doctor's commentary illustrates some of the virtue issues involved:

I saw them on a couple of occasions in the course of a week and struggled with the issue of whether I was 'being taken for a ride' or 'sold a yarn' simply in order to keep the boy out of jail, but managed to satisfy myself that I had a really important social role here, i.e. as someone whose voice might be respected by the court and also almost certainly as the only middle-class figure who had maintained any consistent contact or built up any complex knowledge of this family over two decades. So I have written to the court in terms that make it clear that, while I am no sucker, I do genuinely think that there is a chance that this boy's breach of his Community Service Order represented a 'rock bottom' for him and that a jail sentence could dig the pit irretrievably deeper, while one last chance might help him to climb out of it permanently. (His brother has not only provided accommodation for him, but has also organised some employment.) One aspect of the virtue issue is that I had to struggle with myself over whether I was giving this boy 'an unfair advantage' over the tens of thousands of other juveniles in this situation, who do not happen to have known the same GP for 20 years, but I decided that, on moral grounds, I should certainly not let such a utilitarian consideration inhibit my preparedness to go out on a limb for this lad.

This commentary raises the issues of practical wisdom defined in Hypothesis 3 – the need to make a wise judgment and to assess both one's own capacities and the motivation of the person asking for the help before deciding what to do.

Truth-telling, emphasised in this story, is an important virtue for society to function well,[18] particularly for those in authority whose voice is respected. The virtuous practitioner therefore has a responsibility not merely to say what he or she believes to be true, but to avoid being persuaded to massage the truth for the benefit of an individual patient.

This story supports Hypothesis 4 as, once the request has been posed, to do nothing is to act and Hypothesis 5, that benevolence and courage are particularly important since again acting involves going out on a limb to some degree and being prepared to take part of the blame if things go wrong. Although, as the doctor says, this is not particularly an issue of (distributive) justice, truth-telling can be seen as an element of this virtue for to go beyond the bounds of what the doctor in conscience considers to be the truth would in a sense be unjust.

Conclusion

The method

Considering these stories has demonstrated first that the method has potential. The exploration of real examples of challenges faced by doctors seems to reveal insights into the personal qualities doctors need to flourish.

The concepts of the doctor being called to act as wise friend or good neighbour, which arise directly from the stories discussed above, have to my knowledge not been previously explored.

The richness of the insights that can be gained from exploring stories like these is surprising. I have only considered four stories here, out of more than 80 collected on that one study day. Just as in qualitative research a topic can usually be fully explored by examining the experiences of 15 or 20 people in depth, so here it seems likely that careful examination of a comparatively small number of stories will enable us to develop a fairly detailed characterisation of the virtuous practitioner. Obviously, to test the hypotheses generated above thoroughly (which resemble to some extent Hursthouse's concept of v-rules,[19] generally applicable principles based on a virtue ethics analysis) it would be necessary to consider far more stories than is possible in this short chapter.

The philosophical exploration of these stories has been done by solitary reflection. In future work, it may be more productive to involve a group in an iterative process, collecting stories, exploring their implications and then taking the hypotheses generated back to the group for further exploration and for further stories against which to test them. (Story 3 was generated in response to a request for stories about boundaries, a limited example of this approach.)

The virtues of the GP

The main conclusion from these stories is that at the boundaries doctors may find themselves called upon to act as friends or as good neighbours rather than in a professional role. The virtuous doctor will be flexible and compassionate, not limiting themselves to a formally professional role, and will act in these other roles with courage, temperance and justice as appropriate. Deciding when and how to do so requires considerable practical wisdom. This is part of being not just a virtuous doctor but a virtuous human being.

Being a doctor does not mean that you are not also human – something that traditional approaches to medical ethics tend sometimes to overlook. These stories show how doctors face moral challenges similar to those faced by other people. This observation is self-evident when made, yet strangely given little attention in medical ethics literature.

The research group was deliberately composed of GPs who seemed to be flourishing, in order to obtain stories from that perspective. A psychologist was included to bring other skills to the group, but the fact that he contributed a story that in the event provided some useful insights suggests that (as we might expect) many of the virtues are common to the various primary care professions. Nurses, receptionists, physiotherapists, counsellors, midwives, health visitors – all may be called upon to act as wise friend or good neighbour.

Medical education and the training of other health professionals encourages students to suppress their natural human response to suffering either overtly through exhortations not to get too involved or covertly through the modelling of detachment by teachers and senior members of the profession. The very nature of the course, which traditionally starts with the dissection of a human corpse and proceeds through a detailed study of the human body conceived as a machine, tends to encourage this detachment. Over-involvement can be disabling and is a real danger, but GPs have long recognised that under-involvement – building a wall between yourself and the patient – is neither practical nor effective. The work of the Balint movement[20] and more recently the medical humanities movement[21] has emphasised this. Temperance and practical wisdom in reaching a virtuous balance (a golden mean?) are called for.

This virtue ethics discussion demonstrates that drawing excessively rigid boundaries around the medical role inhibits the doctor from growing and developing as a human being. It would have been possible in all the stories for the doctor to claim that this was not part of his or her job description, but to do so would be neither admirable nor contribute to his or her flourishing as a human being. Responding positively and successfully to difficult situations and situations of need is very satisfying to the doctor concerned. The satisfaction of overcoming the difficulty and the awareness of having been courageous and perceptive (and right!) are part of the 'internal goods' of medical practice,[22] not just a means to achieving them.

In all the stories above the outcome is either positive or unknown. But what if it does not go right? What if the adoption had gone wrong, the dog had been run over outside the doctor's house, the young offender committed manslaughter while on bail? Despite the best efforts of the doctor to apply his or her practical wisdom, there will be cases where they step out of their core medical role with disastrous consequences. This is no argument for not acting virtuously, but what are the virtues needed to flourish in these situations? This empirical question needs to be explored in future work.

The concept of the doctor playing different roles that require different virtues and a different sort of response is valuable not only in helping us to characterise the virtuous practitioner but also in helping the doctor decide what to do in specific situations. It does not, of course, provide an automatic set of answers – this is not the nature of virtue ethics – but it does provide a framework that doctors can use to help them approach a variety of different situations.

The separation and differences between the roles should not be overemphasised. The virtues required of the good neighbour and the wise friend are similar to those needed to succeed in the more core medical roles of the doctor, offering clinical judgments or making rationing decisions. This is, after all, what one would expect – although there are differences in the virtues required of different roles, since they pose different challenges to the people playing them.[23] Our common humanity means that the virtues of different roles are closer to each other than any of them is to vice.

The question of how doctors should act at the boundaries of their role is not the only problem influencing medical morale or public confidence in the medical profession. It is probably not even the most important one. But I think the discussion above shows how a narrative-based, virtue ethics can help us explore this question in a way that is helpful to addressing both our problems. By providing doctors with a framework within which to understand how to act virtuously at the boundaries of their role, the tension that they experience is likely to be lessened and that may contribute to their flourishing. By examining stories in which doctors face and deal with such issues, successfully as in the stories discussed above and perhaps equally catastrophically in others, we can characterise the virtues needed for a good outcome in similar situations to the benefit of both the practitioner and the public. The statements in the last two sentences, of course, pose yet more hypotheses to be tested in future work, underlining that the work described in this chapter is a beginning, not an end.

Thanks are due to those who took part in the research seminar (who to protect patient confidentiality cannot be named). The stories are quoted essentially as reported by seminar participants, but some circumstantial details have been changed to safeguard the anonymity of patients.

References

1 Beauchamp TL, Childress JF. *Principles of Biomedical Ethics*. 4th ed. Oxford: Oxford University Press; 1994.

2 General Medical Council. *Duties of a Doctor*. London: GMC: 1995. http://www.gmc-uk.org/standards/standards_frameset.htm

3 Aristotle. *Ethics*. Thompson JAK, translator. Harmondsworth: Penguin; 1955, revised edn 1976.

4 Aquinas, St Thomas. *Summa Theologica*. Cambridge: Cambridge University Press; 1990, Latin original and English translation.

5 MacIntyre A. *After Virtue – a study in moral theory*. 2nd ed. London: Duckworth & Co; 1985.

6 Hursthouse R. *Applying Virtue Ethics – study guide*. (Open University course A432.) Buckingham: Open University Press; 2000.

7 Nussbaum M, Sen A. *The Quality of Life*. Oxford: Clarendon Press; 1993.

8 Hursthouse R. *Ibid*.

9 Illich I. *Limits to Medicine*. Harmondsworth: Penguin; 1975.

10 Kennedy I. *Unmasking Medicine* (Reith Lectures 1980). Hemel Hempstead: George Allen & Unwin; 1981.

11 *The Bristol Royal Infirmary Inquiry*. http://www.bristol-inquiry.org.uk/index.htm

12 *The Report of The Royal Liverpool Children's Inquiry*. http://www.rlcinquiry.org.uk/

13 *The Shipman Inquiry*. http://www.the-shipman-inquiry.org.uk/home.asp

14 Toon PD. The sovereignty of virtue. *BJGP*. 2002; **52**: 694–5.

15 Toon PD. Defining and cultivating the virtues. *BJGP*. 2002; **52**: 782.

16 Toon PD. What is good general practice? (RCGP Occasional Paper 65.) London: Royal College of General Practitioners; 1994.

17 Aristotle. *Ibid*.

18 Midgely M. *Can't We Make Moral Judgments?* Bristol: Bristol Press; 1991.

19 Hursthouse R. *Virtue Theory and Abortion in Virtue Ethics*. Oxford: Oxford University Press; 1997.

20 Balint M. *The Doctor, his Patient and the Illness*. London: Churchill Livingstone; 1957.

21 Toon PD, Greenhalgh T, Rigby M *et al*. *The Human Face of Medicine* (Apollo Modules 1 and 2 CD Rom). London: BMJ Publishing. 2001.

22 MacIntyre A. *Ibid*.

23 Nussbaum M, Sen A. *Ibid*.

Chapter 7

Interprofessional teamworking: a moral endeavour? An exploration of clinical practice using Seedhouse's ethical grid

Ann King

> Teamwork is essential: it allows you to blame someone else.
>
> Anon

Introduction

Interprofessional working is taken as a given in primary healthcare. Teams are seen as the key to the future of primary care and public health. 'It is evident that community welfare is going to be dependent on good team approaches.'[1] John Horder, former President of the Royal College of General Practitioners (RCGP) has stated that, 'teams benefit patients, clients and professionals alike'.[2] Because the team approach is so fundamental to healthcare, the way people within teams respond to one another is a very important topic for consideration. Team dynamics is a well-established field of interest, but individuals' ethical position in relation to colleagues has tended to be overlooked. The purpose of this chapter is to explore the ethical dimensions of interprofessional working.

How individuals work within a team affects health outcomes as well as having implications for team members themselves. Interprofessional conflict is well researched and documented, although much of it is based on studies in the acute sector. Much has been written about factors that contribute to rivalry and lack of professional collaboration. Children like Victoria Climbie paid the tragic price of poor teamwork. Lord Laming,[3] in his summing up, left little room for misunderstanding as to the importance of teamwork. What we do as team members and how we work together has significant ethical outcomes – 'People's lives and welfare are at risk'[4] and teamwork is therefore an ethical activity.

David Seedhouse's[5] philosophy of health will provide the model for the exploration of the ethics of interprofessional work in this chapter. Seedhouse's work is not without its critics.[6] His views on the relationship between medical ethics and philosophy have attracted attention in the literature. Cassell notes that he does not support a distinction between ethical and non-ethical decisions and thus dismisses a deontological approach to ethical decision-making. Other authors take issue with Seedhouse's claim that there is no distinction between ethical and empirical facts in medicine.[7] But this author supports Seedhouse's approach to include the ordinary and not just the exceptional and dramatic events of medical ethics. Loughlin[8] notes that Seedhouse raises important issues about natural/non-natural distinctions in medicine. The strength of his work is paradoxically the blurring of boundaries between ethics and non-ethics and his inclusion of questions about wider socio-political factors. His work is accessible and applicable to all healthcare professionals and is particularly relevant to the clinical situations being discussed.

Seedhouse informs us that creating health requires ethical commitment and that ethics permeates all aspects of health work. He states that ethical decisions need to be made in context. Henry[9] supports this proposal when he says professionals' reliance on a list of prescriptive rules is no longer tenable and that there is a need for discussion within a wider moral framework. Seedhouse's model provides a framework for in-depth analysis of moral context. He describes health work as a 'moral endeavour' in which health workers commit themselves to a 'powerful moral obligation' over and above the norms expected by society. The powerful moral obligation is explained by Seedhouse's definition of health as that of achieving one's potential (in a given situation). Health work concerns any direct or indirect intervention in others' lives to maximise their potential. Seedhouse views all aspects of health work as a moral endeavour. An example of teamwork as a moral endeavour is presented by Payne,[10] who noted that team functions can have serious and significant implications for human lives. Interprofessional working is an integral part of health work and is therefore part of the moral endeavour. This raises the question as to what the moral obligations that team members owe to one another are.

MacIntyre[11] describes ethics as being concerned with human actions; Seedhouse's theory proposes that ethical actions are 'deliberations about interventions'. Both authors see morality as occurring in a social context, 'Moral life changes as social life changes'. Primary healthcare occurs in diverse and dynamic social situations where staff constantly have to question and re-evaluate situations. Rules, principles and codes are useful aides to ethical deliberations, but are not a simple solution to complex moral questions. Ethical decisions are a matter of degree and consideration for many competing factors. A principal question arises – 'How can I intervene to the highest moral degree'.[12]

The model

Seedhouse's ethical grid (*see* Figure 7.1) is a model for ethical analysis. It consists of four layers, prompting the user to answer the questions raised in each layer. Seedhouse designates each layer by a colour (which are shaded here).

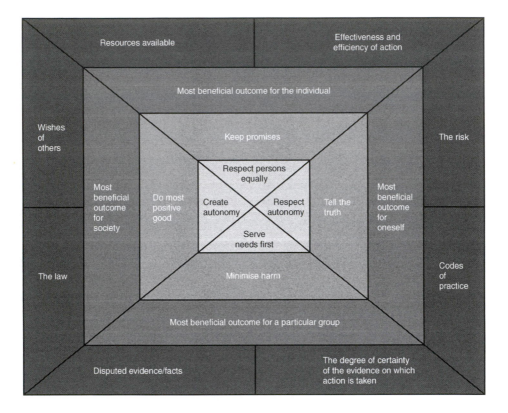

Layer 1 [▨]: Is the intervention going to create autonomy, respect autonomy, treat all persons equally and serve needs first?

Layer 2 [▩]: Is the intervention consistent with moral duties – keeping promises, telling the truth, minimising harm and generating benefit?

Layer 3 [▨]: Is the intervention going to provide the greatest benefit for the greatest number? Furthermore, who will be the benefactors – society, an individual, a group or oneself?

Layer 4 [▩]: Is the intervention likely to be affected by external considerations – resources, the law, risks, disputed evidence or facts and degree of certainty of the evidence on which the action is taken?

Figure 7.1: Simplified ethical grid, reproduced by kind permission of John Wiley & Sons.

This chapter is going to discuss interprofessional teamwork from the premise that it is a moral endeavour, and that teamwork is, directly or indirectly, concerned with interventions that require decisions. The decisions made all have ethical implications; what informs these decisions will be addressed using the model of Seedhouse's ethical grid as a tool to direct discussion and exploration of the wide range of relevant issues.

Definitions

Prior to exploring the ethical dimensions of interprofessional relationships, the terms used need to be clarified. 'Interprofessional' has been chosen from a wide variety of words describing professionals working together: it is best suited, according to Leathard,[13] because 'it refers to interactions between professionals involved, albeit from different backgrounds, but who have the same joint goals in working together.' 'Team' refers to professionals involved in health work, who work together with the common purpose and shared values of meeting community health needs. The team will incorporate the more clearly defined group of staff in GP practices and the wider 'open' teams crossing organisational and professional boundaries. Although much of the material will focus on healthcare professionals (HCPs), it will be pertinent to all interprofessional relationships.

Case studies

The definitions used create a somewhat simplified picture of teams working in primary care. In reality, the situation is complex (*see* Case studies 1 and 2). Primary care teams encompass a wide variety of professionals from different backgrounds and may cover large geographical areas; some team members may never actually see one another, being in contact with their 'virtual' colleagues by e-mail, fax and referral forms or telephone. Computer systems are often incompatible and not all staff have access to them. The team is, in reality, a diverse group of people with different employers, contracts, codes of practice and arguably different agendas. What they should have in common is the shared goal of delivering healthcare. In Case study 1 the outcomes were achieved as a result of good collaborative practice, but this was not so in Case study 2. Yet both occurred within similar contexts. What factors contributed to the team members' ethical decisions?

Case study 1

Mary is a primary school classroom assistant who lives with her partner Paul, a school caretaker. They have two children – Jack aged nearly 4 and Lucy, 5 months. The family has recently moved into the area with Paul's new job. Mary is the main carer for the children and is not employed at present. The family have only been to the practice on a few occasions, to register, for the children's immunisations and for a family planning appointment.

Mary arrived at the well-baby clinic looking strained and tired. Baby Lucy was distressed and her skin was flaky, red and angry; she had a runny nose, sores and scratch marks across her face. Mary explained about her family history of eczema and that she was using a variety of products for her skin. She said she had started using soya milk instead of cow's milk formula the previous day. The Health Visitor (HV) listened to Mary's concerns as she tearfully described her worries and how hard it was to cope with Lucy. The HV suggested that she talk to several colleagues about the issues raised and how best to care for Lucy. The colleagues were the GP, a dietician and the children's hospital-at-home team. It was agreed that the HV would speak to Mary the following afternoon.

The HV contacted the dietician by phone message and a referral form was completed and faxed to her. A copy was sent to the GP. Later on that afternoon, the dietician contacted the HV and discussed Lucy's case, recommending a hydrolysed cow's milk suitable for babies sensitive to cow's milk and highlighted the reasons why soya milk was undesirable. The dietician confirmed she would be contacting Mary by telephone to offer her an appointment and discuss any immediate concerns. The dietician also discussed with the HV whether she was happy to ask the GP to write a prescription. The GP was then contacted and he wrote the prescription while on the phone so that it was available to be collected that evening. The HV then phoned Mary and explained the rationale for the prescription and for not giving soya. The children's hospital-at-home team were contacted by the HV the following morning and they agreed to see Lucy at the beginning of the next week and that they would make contact with Mary, liaise with the GP and give advice on immediate skin care.

> **Case study 2**
>
> Mr Khan has a venous ulcer that requires daily dressings, which until recently were done every day except Sunday by the practice nurse. The practice management team made a decision that they could no longer provide the resources to do dressings on Saturdays.
>
> Mr Khan was referred to the district nursing service, which felt irritated at doing a job that the GP practice should do. District nurses did the dressings for several Saturdays until their managers decided that they could only do dressings for the housebound.
>
> Mr Khan was advised to attend the walk-in service, which involved a car drive from his home and expensive car parking fees. He was then advised, after having his dressings done on several occasions, that chronic wound management was not the remit of the service and that getting his dressings done had depended on the goodwill of staff on duty. The staff felt that they should not be used to 'fill in' for an under-staffed district nursing service. Mr Khan did not want to go all the way into town on the off-chance that he might get his dressings done.
>
> He is now no longer attempting to have his wound dressed on Saturdays and feels angry and upset, especially on Mondays when the wound takes longer to dress and is much more uncomfortable. No one person has personally explained the situation to Mr Khan or taken responsibility for a more positive outcome.

Layer 1 analysis

Layer 1 of the model raises the question of how any chosen intervention will create and/or respect autonomy, treat people equally and serve their needs. The case studies above clearly show the difference between enhanced (Mary) and compromised (Mr Khan).

What is perhaps less clear is that the results may have been mirrored in the staff involved. In Case study 1, the staff worked collaboratively, 'working together to achieve something which neither agency could achieve alone'.[14] Those involved may well have felt a sense of satisfaction as they worked to fulfil their potential as professionals. Dixon and Sweeney[15] discuss how positive relationships are good for health. While they direct their comments to doctor–patient relationships, their findings are relevant to healthcare professionals themselves. They elaborate that healthy interactions are not simply about exchanging information but 'connectedness', where one not only takes part in a conversation but develops an awareness and recognition of the contribution one makes. Being connected allows patients to make sense of their experience and could equally apply to team members gaining appreciation of their own or others' roles. Connecting will result in respecting and creating autonomy in others.

In Case study 2, the staff did not connect, or even communicate, effectively. The various groups withdrew from any potential moral obligation; although they did exercise their autonomy this was at the expense of others. Much research has been done which confirms that this is not unusual. Wicks' thesis,[16] undertaken in a hospital setting, found a lack of respect by doctors for nurses' autonomy. Stein's classic study[17] showed how both actors neither respected nor attempted to create autonomy in the other; they perpetuated their learnt roles.

An essential component of autonomy is integrity, which is 'to develop an internally consistent and incorrupt set of beliefs' and 'a wholeness and solidarity of self that signifies individuality'.[18] Integrity appears to present particular problems for nurses. According to Mitchelle,[18] it is sacrificed to meet medical agendas and nurses almost always experience conflict with physicians because their interprofessional relationships are often in conflict with the nurse–patient relationship. Such a situation results in a lack of coherence between what a nurse feels he or she should do and what he or she actually does. This, of course, could be experienced by any member of the team. Did any professional feel this when they withdrew their services from Mr Khan? To ignore or override another's integrity and therefore their autonomy is to behave unethically.[19]

Hare[20] argues that 'it is a characteristic of moral principles that they cannot be overridden' and from this we can conclude that no one member of the interprofessional team can claim a higher order of moral principles over another. However, literature suggests that dominant and powerful professionals fail to recognise their colleagues' moral principles as having equal status to their own. Integrity of individuals and the team as a whole depends on cooperative interdependent relationships between the parts of the whole.[21] Brown *et al*[22] proposed a means of putting this into practice using the 'Alt White collaborative model', which is based on mutual trust in a non-hierarchical system of communication and responsibility. Integrity and autonomy would be essential components for teams using this approach.

Layer 2 analysis

Layer two of the model has a deontological basis; the broad question concerns duties and moral obligation. Initially this layer would seem straightforward; the answer found in the HCPs' codes of conduct. Codes 'represent an articulated statement of the role morality of the member of the profession'[23] and 'provide an explicit benchmark of expected conduct'.[24] Further analysis produces a more complex and less clear picture.

Both the General Medical Council's (GMC)[25] and the Nursing and Midwifery Council's[26] codes and principles refer to 'duties'. Kendrick[27] states that the central principles are evident in today's codes and the traditional notion of duty continues to inform practice. Kant believed that all people have intrinsic worth, thereby requiring respect; that individuals should not be used as a means to an end, but are ends in their own right; and that people are part of community in which each person is of equal worth as a moral decision maker. These sentiments are evident in our current professional codes.

The principles of respect and intrinsic worth of the individual are evident throughout the codes but in reference to professional patient–client relationships. There is much less said about the duties owed between professionals. Doctors and nurses are told they must have respect for colleagues' skills and expertise. Nurses are required to work cooperatively within teams that incorporate patients, carers and family, indicating that all parties have intrinsic worth. The GMC notes that healthcare is increasingly provided by multidisciplinary teams and interestingly advises, 'make sure that your patients and colleagues understand your professional status and specialty, your role and responsibilities in the team'; it does not indicate a need to understand others' roles. Arguably, the GMC guidelines seem less concerned with collaboration and more with maintaining a powerful position within the team. In Case study 1, Mary was included as part of the team, her opinion was sought and she was fully involved and informed. The requirements of the codes were upheld. In Case study 2, the code was meaningless as no one engaged with anyone else and did not respect or cooperate with colleagues.

Many authors note the limitations of codes, but recognise them as starting points for moral considerations. As a development from codes, the use of the principles emerged and the most often cited, of Beauchamp and Childress,[28] are beneficence, non-maleficence, respect for autonomy and justice. Seedhouse feels strongly that while these principles seem superficially to be a self-evident truth, they achieve little in moral analysis because they frequently compete and there is no model for deciding priority. Putting criticism aside, these principles would appear to be relevant to healthcare, where professionals should benefit clients, avoid harm, respect autonomy and be seen to be just.

Much of the research literature indicates that these principles are not applied to interprofessional relationships within teams. Powerful professions dominate at the expense of others and team members do not respect their colleagues' autonomy, resulting in harm to others' self-confidence, resources not being allocated fairly and arguably little evidence of benefit to all team members. In Case study 2, the groups served their own interests. This could be described as a benefit to each group and, as all groups withdrew their services, a form of equality existed. The groups exercised autonomy to withdraw services, respect for other members did not occur and harm occurred to the client and indirectly to the professionals' reputations. So, while it could be argued that three out of the four principles were applied, the outcome was probably morally unacceptable and fell short of being a moral endeavour.

The codes, as part of the moral endeavour for health, were useful but limited in their direction to achieve the highest possible level of morality. Team members need to do more than cooperate and/or respect colleagues. They need to incorporate the strategies discussed in Layer 1 by enhancing autonomy, connecting and working collaboratively so that the ethical principles discussed in Layer 2 become alive and relevant. An integrated non-hierarchical team, which respected and created autonomy in its members while valuing awareness of each individual's level of experience and learning needs, would most probably have naturally incorporated the principles outlined.

Layer 3 analysis

The next layer is not concerned with individual rights or duties but with goals and outcomes. It comes under the broad umbrella of consequentalism, which 'is a label offered to theories holding that actions are right or wrong according to the balance of their good or bad consequences'.[29] This school of thought had its origins in the 18th century, first with Bentham and later, Mill. Among other things, Bentham focused on pleasure versus pain when weighing consequences – so called 'hedonistic utilitarianism'. Mill refined the theory, broadening the concept of benefit. It seems very logical and appealing to do the greatest good for the majority until one considers it a little further. Is it justice to improve the lives of the majority by ignoring the needs of a minority? How can you equate disadvantage, suffering and possibly harm with other people's wellbeing? This raises questions. Who is making these decisions? Are they going to benefit themselves and if so, is that acceptable? What if the majority desires something that is considered immoral? What happens to individual rights, sanctity of life and the principle of justice?

Utilitarians themselves were aware of some of the limitations and difficulties the theory presented and this engendered several different types of utilitarianism. Act-utilitarianism aims to produce the greatest balance of good over evil, i.e. actions that are justified by the end product of utility. This approach could produce problems within healthcare organisations because one person's view of the greatest utility may not be shared by others. Rule-utilitarianism identifies rules that are justified by utility and conforming to the rule makes the act preferable.

Utilitarianism appears to lend itself readily to patients and much less to interprofessional teams. The concept of team already discussed would indicate that all members benefit from their common goal and shared values. Reality indicates a different picture; research on interprofessional teams indicates that different professional groups within teams do not feel that they are valued and autonomous members of the team. Does this matter if a team is delivering what is expected? Mitchelle[30] quotes Bernard Williams: 'utilitarianism cannot hope to make sense, at any level of integrity'. However, Mitchelle herself counters this with a discussion about the consequences to patient care of staff whose integrity is jeopardised. Case study 1 illustrates how utility could be achieved on different levels. The staff involved respected each other's roles, which in itself produces utility: staff who function optimally are likely to deliver better care and hence greater utility.

It is possible that teams will function so as to maximise utility for themselves at the expense of their moral endeavour in healthcare delivery, Mr Khan being a case in point. The individual groups within the wider team acted to increase their own benefit by refusing to do the dressings on weekends for what were considered to be good reasons. Their individual interests were protected to the detriment of Mr Khan, who was powerless to change or challenge the situation. So while in numerical terms the greater number gained, the outcome was morally unacceptable. There could well be a situation where healthcare professionals may make decisions to protect themselves at a cost to the patient that is morally acceptable and correct. For example, an emergency situation may present such a level of risk to staff that they have to evacuate and leave the patient. HCPs do not have a moral obligation to risk life and limb for patients – utility would not be served by dead or maimed professionals.

Seedhouse recommends that Layer 3 is used to ask who is being considered for benefit. Is it an individual in the team, one's self, a group or does it have wider considerations for society? Singer[31] describes utilitarianism as being a minimal position or a first base. He believes it to be a good starting point, but one that should be abandoned if there is good evidence that other moral rules can provide more persuasive answers. Seedhouse suggests that Layer 3 should not be used alone but in conjunction with other aspects of the grid. Layer 3 allows the issue of who is benefiting to be examined and the morality to be questioned.

Layer 4 analysis

The final layer of the model helps to highlight some of the moral complexities facing professionals within teams and the factors that play a part in the interventions available to the moral agent. Layer 4 asks for consideration to be given to the wider issues that influence interprofessional interactions and subsequently their interventions for health. Seedhouse believes that insufficient attention is given to these wider issues when discussing healthcare ethics. This layer questions a team's interactions and interventions within the wider influences of society.

Ethical decisions are not made in a vacuum but take place within cultures with their own moral agenda. MacIntyre,[32] when discussing the historic development of ethical theory, makes it clear that morals are both culturally and historically changeable. Moral behaviour is open to negotiation within society and undergoes changes over time.

Both case studies indicate that within the health service there are discrepancies in team functions and that moral behaviour can be significantly different among teams with supposedly shared values and objectives. The moral endeavour for health is not static or uniformly achieved; it is constantly challenged by numerous factors within and outside of the healthcare team.

The nature of professional boundaries

Greenwall and Walby[33] undertook a study investigating the nature of professional boundaries within an acute hospital. Many of their findings have relevance to primary care, principally because professionals in the community have been trained and socialised in their professional roles within the acute sector. The main themes that are evident in the work are historic, organisational, role and gender. These broad themes will be used as a basis for discussion within the context of Layer 4. They are not clear cut and all interlink.

Historic changes have left their imprint on today's practices and, despite greater understanding and debate, still appear to haunt contemporary beliefs about healthcare practice. The historic context will only be briefly discussed to highlight how some present-day issues developed. Although history can be interpreted in different ways, it cannot be changed; however, it can indicate the depth of a situation and how entrenched it may be.

Nursing has traditionally been a female profession, originally formed from a body of women from poor or religious backgrounds. From the 19th century onwards the nursing profession recruited women from upper- and middle-class backgrounds, following Florence Nightingale's overhaul of the profession. The role of the nurse has remained the same. Nurses serve the same role as the women in the patriarchal family, where the man is dominant and the female is supportive and caring. These virtues of a good woman have been directly transferred to the virtues of a good nurse.

Ackroyd[34] notes that as nursing was almost exclusively associated with being a female occupation, it was viewed less favourably and as a result is poorly paid. Nightingale established training schools for suitable women that perpetuated the hierarchical divisions between nursing and medicine. She is quoted as saying, 'for nursing is the skilled servant of medicine and training has to make her not servile but loyal to the medical orders and authority'. Both historically and today, nurses have been denied positions of authority. Aneurin Bevan refused to have nurses on the newly-formed health service management committees; he felt they had no place there. Today nurses and other professionals are represented on the professional executive committees of primary care trusts, but questions remain about the ratio of medical to non-medical professionals, selection criteria and proportionality.

The development of a profession has already been alluded to. It is a subject that has attracted a great deal of attention, some of which sheds light on the interactions of modern team members with each other. The term 'professional' has been used throughout this chapter to refer to all trained staff. However, controversially, it has been argued[35] that while GPs are professionals, other HCPs are semi-professionals.

By examining the definitions, we are able to see the potential for conflict in practice. The sociologist, Freidson[36] describes a profession as 'an occupation which has assumed a dominate position on a division of labour, so that it gains control over the determination of the substance of its own work'. He proposed that once a profession has achieved this position, it can be considered to be a reliable authority.

The semi-professionals, in contrast to the professionals, undergo shorter training, do not have self-determination in their work, lack full autonomy, and are granted fewer privileges and less status. Greenwall and Walby's[37] study would appear to support these differences in that they found nurses working in hospital teams to be much more management-led, working to prescribed guidance and protocols, in contrast to doctors who were more independent and self-determined. The authors noted that each of these modes of working could have negative implications for teamwork.

Much criticism has been levelled at the professions that have become so powerful, enabling self-regulation and self-interest to the extent that they no longer respond to the needs of their clients. Rather, they impose their own agenda on the users of the service and thus do not fulfil the key role of being a professional serving the client. An alternative approach to delivering care is suggested by Toon's[38] compassionate practitioner, based on the ethics of virtue as defined by St Thomas Aquinas, who claimed that 'the habit or disposition of acting rightly according to right reason' brings into focus the care of the client. Toon proposes that application of the virtues of faith, fortitude, temperance, charity and hope can change the balance of power, encourage inclusion and also limit litigation. The application of Toon's recommendation would provide a more inclusive definition of 'professional', which is truly responsive to the needs of both patient and colleagues.

The HCPs in Case study 2 served their own (and arguably legitimate) needs, but by failing to resolve who should do the dressings, they imposed their own reality on an individual who had no form of redress. Some light may possibly be shed on their course of action by Schön's[39] famous work on 'the reflective practitioner'. He claims that high degrees of specialisation can lead to parochial narrowing of vision, which results in failure to see the whole person. This failure, if perpetuated, can lead to burnout and boredom, which will both undermine any attempts within teams to respond to health needs. Professionals working in a team need to develop awareness of how the team is responding to the demands on the service.

Gender is a subject that occurs as a theme in Greenwall and Walby's[40] study; it is not a self-contained category, but is entwined with historic and professional developments. It plays a significant role in organisational structure. Gender was probably the single most important factor in the emergence of the occupation of nursing. Many women practise medicine, as men practise nursing, yet the gender-based games described in Stein's[41] doctor–nurse game still resonate. The nurse takes on the female role of manipulating the dominant player, medicine, which adopts the masculine role. Both sets of actors avoid open communication and the collaboration recommended by Brown et al.[42]

Why do gender games continue? Kendrick[43] suggests that it is in part due to nurses operating from a different power base. The power base will be weaker as a result of nurses generally coming from less well-educated backgrounds and their training being much less scientific and therefore considered to be less objective. Oakley[44] notes that research indicates that those in subordinate groups are socialised to be dependent and sensitive to the needs of the dominant group, who are more independent and focused on their own welfare.

Organisational structure is probably the most significant factor in inhibiting the realisation of health work as a moral endeavour. It can prevent the creation of autonomy and could well be described as 'dwarfing' individuals. The results will be silent and unlabelled but very noticeable if searched for.

Henry[45] states that gender issues in organisations cannot be changed from within, which could in part explain why the system is not challenged by nurses. The organisational structure reinforces gender division and could be said to precipitate conflict. Freeman and Miller[46] state that one of the reasons teams are unable to work effectively is because of organisational features. Mitchelle[47] describes two competing, and in many respects incompatible, models of delivering healthcare: the mission model and the sensitive model. The former is medically-orientated and managed from top down, and nurses are essential participants in meeting the aims and goals of the model. In contrast, the sensitive model is structured from bottom up to meet the multiple needs of patients. Despite the mantra of meeting individual patients' needs, much moral conflict experienced by nurses results from a clash between the two models. Nurses, according to Mitchelle, are rarely included in moral decision-making, indicating that one professional group is assumed to have a higher order of moral principles over their colleagues.

Conclusion

Interprofessional working is taken as a self-evident truth, yet as Ovretveit[48] notes there is a lack of progress in developing effective interprofessional teams. By using the modified ethical grid the extent and implication of this for both successful and failed interprofessional work can be seen to have far-reaching consequences. The examples discussed highlight how health work as a moral endeavour may increase and potentiate individuals' autonomy or how both professionals' and patients' integrity is violated and compromised. De Raeve[49] raises the important need for healthcare institutions to stop ignoring the moral issues arising from interprofessional conflict. Until the ethical dimensions of interprofessional working relationships are acknowledged, recognised and examined, the full moral endeavour of health work will fail to be achieved.

References

1 Maude A. The power of partnership. *Public Health News*. 1 November 2004.

2 Horder J. Foreword. In: Leathard A, ed. *Interprofessional Collaboration: from policy to practice in health and social care*. London: Routledge; 2003.

3 Lord Laming. (2001) *Laming Inquiry: Victoria Climbie inquiry*. 2001; http://www.victoria-climbie-inqury.org.uk

4 Payne M. *Team Work in Multi-Professional Care*. Basingstoke: Macmillan Press; 2000.

5 Seedhouse D. *Ethics; The Heart of Healthcare*. New York: John Wiley & Sons; 1988.

6 Hill D. Response to David Seedhouse's 'commitment to health: a shared ethical bond between professions'. *J Interprofessional Care*. 2002; **16**(3): 261–4; Kottow MH. In defence of medical ethics. *J Med Ethics*. 1999; **25**: 340–3; Cassell J. Against ethics: opening the can of worms. *J Med Ethics*. 1998; **24**(February): 8–12.

7 Toon P. Medical ethics: a brief response to Seedhouse. *J Med Ethics*. 1995; **21**: 47–8.

8 Loughlin M. Arguments at cross-purposes: moral epistemology and medical ethics. *J Med Ethics*. 2005; **28**: 28–32.

9 Henry C. Professional ethics and organisational change. In: Soothill K, Macky L, Webb C, eds. *Interprofessional Relations in Healthcare*. London: Arnold; 1995.

10 Payne M. *Ibid*.

11 MacIntyre A. *A Short History of Ethics: a history of moral philosophy from the Homeric age to the twentieth century*. London: Routledge; 1993.

12 Seedhouse D. *Ibid*.

13 Leathard A, ed. *Interprofessional Collaboration: from policy to practice in health and social care*. London: Routledge; 2003.

14 Ovretveit J, Mathias P, Thompson T, eds. *Interprofessional Working of Health and Social Care*. London: Macmillan; 1997.

15 Dixon M, Sweeney K. *The Human Effects in Medicine: theory, research and practice*. Oxford: Radcliffe Medical Press; 2000.

16 Wicks D. *Nurses and Doctors at Work: rethinking professional boundaries*. Buckingham: Open University Press; 1998.

17 Stein LI. The doctor–nurse game. *Arch Gen Psychiatry*. 1967; **16**: 699–703.

18 Mitchelle C. Integrity in interprofessional relationships. In: Agida G, ed. *Responsibility in Healthcare*. Dordrecht: Kluwer; 1982.

19 Brown J, Stewart M, Weston W, eds. *Challenges and Solutions in Patient-Centered Care: a case book*. Oxford: Radcliffe Medical Press; 2002.

20 Hare R. Integrity in interprofessional relationships. In: Agida G, ed. *Responsibility in Healthcare*. Dordrecht: Kluwer; 1982.

21 Brown J *et al*. *Ibid*.

22 Brown J *et al*. *Ibid*.

23 Beauchamp TC, Childress JF. *Principles of Biomedical Ethics*. Oxford: Oxford University Press; 1994.

24 Wall A. Some ethical issues arising from interprofessional working. In: Leathard A, ed. *Interprofessional Collaboration: from policy to practice in health and social care*. London: Routledge; 2003.

25 General Medical Council. *Good Medical Practice*. London: GMC; 2001.

26 Nursing and Midwifery Council. *Codes of Professional Conduct*. London: Nursing and Midwifery Council; 2002.

27 Kendrick K. Codes of professional conduct and the dilemmas of professional practice. In: Soothill K, Mackay L, Webb C. *Interprofessional Relations in Healthcare*. London: Arnold; 1995.

28 Beauchamp TC, Childress JF. *Ibid*.

29 Kendrick K. *Ibid*.

30 Mitchelle C. *Ibid*.

31 Singer P. *Practical Ethics*. Cambridge: Cambridge University Press; 1994.

32 MacIntyre A. *Ibid*.

33 Greenwall J, Walby S. *Medicine and Nursing: professions in a changing health service*. London: Sage Publications; 1994.

34 Ackroyd S. Nurses, management and morale: a diagnosis of decline in the NHS hospital service. In: Soothill K, Mackay L, Webb C. *Interprofessional Relations in Healthcare*. London: Arnold; 1995.

35 Etizliomi A. *The Semi-Professionals and their Organisation*. New York: Free Press; 1969.

36 Freidson E. Profession of medicine: a study of the sociology of applied knowledge. In: Mackay L. *Classic Texts in Healthcare*. Oxford: Butterworth-Heinemann; 1998.

37 Greenwall J, Walby S. *Ibid*.

38 Toon PD. Towards a philosophy of general practice: a study of the virtuous practitioner. *Occasional Chapters*. 1999; **78**(April): ii–viii, 1–69.

39 Schön D. *The Reflective Practitioner: how professionals think in action*. New York: Basic Books; 1983.

40 Greenwall J, Walby S. *Ibid*.

41 Stein LI. *Ibid*.

42 Brown J *et al*. *Ibid*.

43 Kendrick K. Nurses and doctors: a problem of partnership. In: Soothill K, Mackay L, Webb C. *Interprofessional Relations in Healthcare*. London: Arnold; 1995.

44 Oakley A. The importance of being a nurse. In: Mackay L. *Classic Texts in Healthcare*. Oxford: Butterworth-Heinemann; 1998.

45 Henry O. Professional ethics and organisational change. In: Soothill K, Mackay L, Webb C. *Interprofessional Relations in Healthcare*. London: Arnold; 1995.

46 Freeman M, Miller C. Clinical teamwork: the impact of policy on collaborative practice. In: Leathard A, ed. *Interprofessional Collaboration: from policy to practice in health and social care*. London: Routledge; 2003.

47 Mitchelle C. *Ibid*.

48 Ovretveit J. *Ibid*.

49 de Raeve L. Medical authority and nursing integrity. *J Med Ethics*. 2002; **28**: 353–7.

Chapter 8

Complexity, guidelines and ethics

Jim Price and Deborah Bowman

> A man's ethical behaviour should be based effectually on sympathy, education, and social ties.[1]
>
> Albert Einstein

Introduction

Clinical decision-making both for the novice and experienced professional is often difficult. Judgments have to be made in a complex environment, balancing the needs, wants and knowledge of the patient with the best available evidence. Decisions are taken in the context of a professional relationship, which may differ in the degree of trust and respect between the two parties, as well as in their belief systems. In effect every clinical encounter is unique, and ethical and moral principles to guide these actions are both needed and unavoidable. The inherent uncertainty, particularly of primary care, renders the reconciliation of individual circumstance, complexity, evidence and ethical decision-making particularly challenging.

Clinical guidelines are now often developed (although not necessarily used)[2] to help this complex decision-making process, but because the interaction of the clinician, the patient and the guideline is complex, and the outcome sometimes unpredictable, ethical principles are important in determining the outcome of this interaction. It has been suggested that doctors new to family medicine may have different attitudes towards clinical guidelines.[3] Ethics should, of course, provide the framework in which all of clinical practice occurs. However, when decisions are complex and involve inherent vulnerabilities that may be discomforting, attention to ethics provides a device by which to scrutinise them.

This chapter discusses the ethical aspects of clinical decision-making, using the consultation and clinical guidelines as a springboard to dive into the whirlpool of complexity theory. While top-down ethics might frame expected behaviour, it is argued that an ethics of complexity, linked closely to moral sensitivity, arises locally in a continual process as an emergent and relational property of a complex system, such as a doctor–patient–guideline interaction.

Complexity and the consultation

Consider first a scenario from a typical GP training practice in the NHS.

The GP registrar (GPR) was new. She was doing her first surgeries after an introductory month. The patient had been referred from the practice nurse after three readings of high blood pressure, which were confirmed with 24-hour ambulatory pressure monitoring. The consultation was difficult: a middle-aged, obese man with few other risk factors for cardiovascular disease, other than a family history. The GPR explained that it was important to treat the patient's hypertension and referred, in her explanation, to the 'evidence' that untreated hypertension contributes to premature disease and even death. The patient challenged the GPR, saying, 'You doctors are always coming up with "evidence" for something you do or don't want us to do, and it changes every five minutes.'

The patient declined the GPR's advice of treatment. The GPR was uncertain how to proceed, but managed to bring the consultation to a rather unsatisfactory end with a review planned. The GPR felt uneasy and later asked her trainer about the consultation. The GPR and trainer were discussing the case:

GPR: I really didn't know what to do with this patient. The NICE [National Institute for Health and Clinical Excellence; previously National Institute for Clinical Excellence] guidelines are clear but he was very reluctant to take any drug treatment. His BP was high and I wanted to do the best for him, but at the same time I didn't want to jeopardise our relationship and I wasn't sure how to proceed.

Trainer: Why do you think he wouldn't take the tablets?

GPR: He seemed to be well informed, but mentioned that his father had died soon after starting treatment for hypertension. I don't think he really believed me when I said that taking tablets was likely to reduce his risk of stroke or heart attack. He said he didn't believe in 'evidence', since every patient is different, and had also read on the Internet that there's disagreement between BP guidelines.

Continued

Trainer:	What issues does this raise for you?
GPR:	Well ... treating blood pressure should be fairly straightforward and it's important to follow the guidelines. After all, we know that poorly controlled hypertension puts patients at unnecessary risk. I certainly didn't expect the patient to know about conflicting guidelines or react as he did. I don't want to alienate him, but I need to convince him why it matters that he gets good treatment, don't I?
Trainer:	What do you think about the NICE guidelines?
GPR:	I felt very anxious, particularly when he wouldn't follow the guideline and it made me realise how difficult some clinical encounters can be even when the situation at first seems straightforward.

As a prelude to a discussion of ethics in complex systems, it is useful to define what complexity means in this context. Complexity theory has developed into an influential worldview or meta-theory, originating in mathematics and chaos theory, but gradually pervading diverse fields. It has indeed been hailed as the 'new science'[4] in the biophysical arena, as well as competing for the top spot in management science.[5] It offers an explanatory framework for the connectedness of the living world, being a fundamental property of networks, and is perhaps best understood in terms of process, rather than structure.[6] There are many definitions of complex systems. Mitleton-Kelly[7] describes 10 generic principles of complex evolving systems, which are summarised below with examples to show how they might apply to the doctor–patient–guideline interaction in the case study.

Ten principles of complex evolutionary systems[8]

1 Connectivity and interdependence

Complex behaviour arises from the interrelationship, interaction and interconnectivity of elements within a system, and between a system and its environment. In a human system, such as a doctor–patient consultation, this means that the behaviour of one individual may affect the other individual and the system. In turn, the contribution of a person in a particular context depends partly on the other individuals within that group – for instance, the input of the wider practice team or the influence of the GP trainer.

2 Coevolution

In biological terms, coevolution means that adaptation by one organism alters the fitness and the fitness landscapes of other organisms. In human systems, coevolution emphasises the relationships between the coevolving entities. Through a complexity lens, it makes no sense to examine the evolution or performance of one individual in isolation – the GPR and patient coevolve.

3 Far from equilibrium; 4 Exploration of the possibility space

Nicolis and Prigogine[9] showed that when a physical or chemical system is pushed away from equilibrium it survives and thrives, while if it remains at equilibrium it dies. The reason is that when far from equilibrium, systems are forced to explore their space of possibilities and this exploration helps them to create new patterns of relationships and different structures. It could be argued that this is how learning and innovation occur: a good model for both the doctor–patient relationship and the GPR–trainer relationship.

5 History

In a social context, the choices that an individual makes partly determine the subsequent path of that individual. Indeed whether an individual perceives there to be a choice or decision to be made at all is a social and value-laden personalised process. Before a decision is made, there are a number of alternatives (which may be understood quite differently by different individuals even if the situation is apparently identical). After the decision is made it becomes part of history and influences the subsequent options open to the individual. Thus the decisions made in one consultation will affect those made in the next. Each patient and each doctor contribute to, and are influenced by, their individual and collective histories in making even commonplace decisions.

6 Feedback

Feedback is how the system remains tuned to its environment and landscape, enabling it to adjust its behaviour. In conditions that are far from equilibrium, change is non-linear; small changes may be amplified and produce exponential change. For example, a throwaway phrase by the doctor can have far-reaching effects on the patient, or vice versa (as in the case study).

7 Path dependence and increasing returns

It has been argued[10] that although conventional economic theory is based on the assumption of diminishing returns, sometimes positive feedback loops magnify a shift and lead to increasing returns. A boom and bust economy is a classical example of this, but one might also see dramatic change in a doctor–patient relationship, with one disagreement or misunderstanding after another leading to a complete breakdown in trust.

8 Self-organisation; 9 Emergence; 10 Creation of new order

Emergent properties arise from the interaction of the elements in the system, and the patterns and new order created could not have been predicted by looking at the behaviour of the individual agents. One cannot understand the whole by breaking it down into its component parts. As Cilliers states,[11] 'a complex system is non-compressible'; therefore, modelling any such system will never be perfect. For example role-plays in GPR teaching will never quite capture the real thing.

Certainty and truth

The impromptu GPR tutorial is probably similar to many that occur daily in GP training practices. The importance of communication in the clinical encounter is obvious and it also highlights the different belief systems sometimes held by doctor and patient. This case also illustrates complexity of ethical decision-making in an apparently straightforward case. The GPR may have felt there should be a 'right way' to proceed: she was using the guidelines to seek certainty, although her quest for certainty in treating the patient may, at least superficially, put her at odds with the ethical principle of autonomy. However, a more rigorous and subtle analysis of the concept of autonomy, coupled with the insights of complexity theory, may offer some new perspectives on the problem.

The quest for certainty and truth is as old as philosophy itself. The debate between realists and constructivists is evident in the writing of Heraclitus. He asserted, 'Upon those who step into the same river different and ever different waters flow down' – a contrast to Plato's belief that 'the Universe really is a motion and nothing else'. This principle of motion, combined with Aristotelian teleology (the tendency towards absolute fulfilment or entelechy), or in other words the urge for self-realisation, provided the context for the challenge of Cartesian dualism and Newtonian mechanics that led to the influential 19th-century

Positivist movement.[12] The latter, despite the seminal critiques offered by writers such as Kuhn,[13] has influenced both ideas about the nature of truth and knowledge (ontology/epistemology) and the education and practice of clinicians. The positivist dependence on rules and principles is evident in ethical thought in the writing of Kant.[14] Currently, the General Medical Council (GMC)[15] arguably continues to equate ethical behaviour predominantly with precepts and rules. In medicine, many clinicians assume that there is one right answer to a medical problem and also one correct way to act. This is resonant of the notion of the 'free descent of ethics from above' (in contrast to the perspective of the 'slow ascent of ethics from below').[16] A complexity perspective favours the latter approach, while acknowledging alternative perspectives.

Certainty in medicine

This positivist backdrop frames biomedicine and therefore influences, albeit not exclusively, the belief system of those who have had a biomedical training.[17] Although clinical and postgraduate training, particularly perhaps in general practice, emphasises the social, interactionist and psychological dimensions of medicine,[18] this work builds on a predominantly positivist base in which the world is presented as ultimately predictable, whereby if we understood all the laws of physics and had enough information, we could know everything. The Cartesian notion of a mechanical universe still pervades medical science and, to some extent, training,[19] despite the nagging of 19th-century Romanticism and the resurgence of holism in the last 100 years, following the shock that 'systems cannot be understood by analysis'.[20] Uncertainty has pervaded physics since Heisenberg,[21] yet physicists still strive to combine quantum and wave theory into the holy grail of a 'theory of everything'.[22] If this search for explanation, consistency and replicable knowledge parallels, even subconsciously, the thinking of the GPR, it begins to become clear why she is struggling with her hypertensive patient and the ambiguity in guidelines.

In common practice, most secondary care physicians continue to work to eliminate uncertainty and primarily act as though there were a cause and effect for the illness of each patient. Although sociologists have explored the ways in which uncertainty pervades even the work of doctors working in specialties as diverse as haematology,[23] surgery,[24] cardiology,[25] genetics[26] and paediatrics,[27] the aim is largely to recreate the clinical encounter to present, if not certainty, at least tolerable uncertainty by providing diagnosis (and treatment) for the patient. Consequently, many tests and investigations are performed in secondary care to minimise clinical uncertainty. In general practice, living with uncertainty goes with the territory, but political forces raise the stakes and some have argued that public expectations have risen,[28] fuelling the drive for certainty even in primary care. In many cases we could be more certain by performing more investigations, and this lies at the heart of the mismatch between demand and resources in the NHS.

The sands also shift. What appears as a fact one-day will be refuted the next. For example, beta-blockers were once contraindicated in heart failure and now they are almost first-line treatment.[29] Such changes further challenge the notion of certainty in medicine. The changing environment is typified in the 'swampy-lowlands' of general practice[30] and is the environment of complexity, where non-linear causality seems rife, where there is a priority of relationships and interconnections above cause and effect, and emergent patterns appear in the interaction between professionals and patients. In the 'swamp', clinical decisions are constantly required and, despite the primacy of patient autonomy and importance of shared decision-making, legal responsibility for these decisions generally resides with the physician. GPs, Berger argues, are constantly balancing the uncertainties of practice with their underlying 'unsatisfied quest for certainty'.[31]

Uncertainty, particularly in primary care, has been the subject of much analysis.[32] Simon[33] uses the concept of 'bounded rationality' as a foundation for decisions where knowledge is limited. For the purposes of considering the GPR and her patient, the challenge is not merely to make a decision in the face of uncertainty, but to make an ethical decision that embraces different values, i.e. for the GPR (with the help of her trainer) to make a 'good enough' decision in a situation where it appears impossible, because of the patient's resistance to treatment, to make what the GPR considers an optimal decision. As Goodman states,[34] 'the embracing of such a view rescues us from the extremes of decision incapacity or inertia on the one side, and winging it on the other'. Bounded rationality resonates with the systems approach adopted by complexity theory where systems are seen as constrained by semi-permeable or fuzzy boundaries.

So can complexity theory help us with decision-making? At one level, it appears the answer might be 'no'. Examining a clinical encounter through the lens of complexity, it is clear that clinical decisions need to be made without having a model or a method that can predict the exact outcome of those decisions. Complexity theory implies that non-linear systems can change suddenly from one state to another non-deterministically, influenced by random individual acts. Thus it is possible for individuals to have profound effects on the future state of the system.

Individuals working as professionals within the system, like the GPR, need to be aware of and comfortable with their capacity for affecting processes; what might be described as moral sensitivity. However, if the GPR is incapable of predicting the state of the future system, how can the imperative to be morally sensitive be anything other than burdensome? Complexity theory proposes that actions have consequences, but those consequences are determined on system levels of which agents never have full knowledge. Therefore, although the GPR in the case is responsible for her own actions, it is unlikely she will affect the system in the way she intended. As Cilliers states, 'A theory of complexity cannot provide us with a method to predict the effects of our decisions, nor the way to predict the future behaviour of the system under consideration.'[35] However, Cilliers goes on to acknowledge that decisions are unavoidable, positively enhance systems and, in the absence of calculation and prediction, demand ethical analysis.

This is key: complexity theory both demands and informs ethical competence. The GPR is not burdened with the requirement that she be morally sensitive because she interacts with each patient and produces unexpected effects, but is empowered by the realisation that unexpected events occur in consultations where values collide, previous histories and experiences meet and unpredicted exchanges take place. She is liberated from the confines of the linear, positivist straight jacket that defines her role as provider of predetermined, universally desirable treatment for hypertension and given permission to consider her role as part of a larger, dynamic and potentially more fruitful process of engagement with the patient.

Thus, as Cilliers argues, an ethical stance is not something imposed on any individual or organisation, but is 'the inevitable result of the inability of a theory of complexity to provide a complete description of all aspects of the system'.[36] The GPR's clinical decisions are made in local semi-bounded systems with her patients (which are themselves nested in larger complex systems within the practice, the PCT, the NHS and beyond). We know the doctor–patient relationship to be of central importance and it can be further elucidated by exploring the relationship of 'self' to 'other', a central feature in recent post-modern discourse.

Post-modernism and otherness

In the case study, the GPR was intensely aware of the difference between her own mindset and that of the patient. Equally, the guidelines were seen as 'out there' and a separate source of propositional or representational knowledge. In the post-modern world, difference is a central concept. Adopting a relational view of complexity theory, difference is important in that relationships between agents in a system define the emergent patterns of behaviour and the self emerges in the interaction of two or more agents, which are codependent and interpenetrative.

Thus post-modernity informs the complexity lens and ethical decision-making because it allows for different interactions and contrasting yet coexistent and dynamic versions of self as the GPR interacts with the patient, her trainer and even the guidelines. The GPR, as a unitary self, is changed by interaction with both the patient and with the guidelines and trainer.

Smith[37] suggests that the role of the GP is 'negotiating understandings, persuading, empowering, supporting and enabling, rather than legislating and controlling'. While this may be the case, the reflexive nature of the relationship is equally important and perhaps only inferred in Smith's notion of the GP's role. The GP does not negotiate, persuade, empower, support and enable as a consistently neutral facilitator, rather the GP herself both affects, and is affected by, each interaction in every consultation. Stacey refers to the 'complex responsive process' of human relating,[38] a view considered by some[39] to be on the 'left wing' of mainstream complexity thinking. The doctor–patient relationship can be seen as a complex responsive process whereby interaction changes both parties on a continual basis and, although bounded by contextual expectations and rules, emergent patterns of behaviour, often novel and surprising, do appear and change the context for the continuing relationship of the two agents. Ethical behaviour may be seen as an emergent and necessary property of the continuing relationship. However, how does this help the GPR who may have learnt that she is part of a system that she both affects and is affected by and therefore requires her to be morally sensitive? In learning to embrace the uncertainty of even routine encounters and question apparently applicable guidelines, how does she use this learning to make the ethical decisions demanded of her?

Fitness

A good starting point for the GPR and her trainer is to scrutinise the purpose of the interaction. What is the system trying (teleologically) to achieve? One view would be that any system is trying to maximally adapt to its environment, i.e. to achieve fitness. The fitness landscape of a complex system may be described as the bounded space in which the complex system operates. Within this landscape, certain patterns and routes are more favourable for the survival of the system in the future, resonating with Darwinian notions of evolutionary niches. The patterns of behaviour emerging in interactions such as that of the doctor–patient relationship might then be viewed as pathways in an ethical landscape.[40] Values become codependent and might flow as rivers and lakes between mountain valleys in a geographical landscape. They will affect (or be dependent upon) each other to a greater or less degree. Values are thus not objects in themselves, they are relationships.[41] As Bateson[42] argues, 'destroy the pattern which connects and you destroy all quality as well'. Thus, the GPR and her trainer must first reflect on the values she has and how these relate to the ultimate moral endeavour of the consultation. However, how does elucidating values contribute to clarity when considering ethics through a complexity lens? The answer lies in the concept of autopoiesis.

Constructivism and ecological thinking

Maturana and Varela[43] coined the term 'autopoiesis' for the Aristotelian notion of 'self-realisation' or 'self-creation'. Autopoiesis refers to the ability of organisms to reproduce themselves as autonomous unities in an inseparable connection ('structural coupling') with their environment. The coexistence of others necessitates an interaction with another in order to 'fit' to the environment. The nature of this interaction 'implies an ethics we cannot evade, an ethics that has its basis in the biological and social structure of human beings, an ethics that puts human reflection right at the core as a constitutive social phenomenon'.[44] The idea of autopoiesis and 'structured coupling' has also been developed and claimed as a paradigm change in social systems theory[45] and legal theory.[46]

This constructivist view of the world, with knowledge as non-representational, is seen as an 'epistemological Odyssean journey between the Scylla monster of representationism and the Charybdis whirlpool of solipsism'.[47]

Sailing this careful course is similar to the journey between moral absolutism (deontology) and moral relativism. The moral absolutist ignores emotions and feelings, whereas moral relativism is sometimes nihilistically situational with the attendant risk that choice depends on convenience, habit or personal taste. In developing an ethical framework to guide choice in clinical decision-making, it is argued that the GPR needs to adopt a model that offers a moral rationale for promoting (as a minimum) human wellbeing. So, how might the patient's wellbeing be best considered by the GPR?

Values and beliefs systems

Despite wanting to promote his wellbeing and health, our GPR realised that her belief system was at variance with that of her patient. Her beliefs interacted (clashed) with those of her patient and the outcome was uncomfortable. Viewing a belief system as a nested system or even as an autonomous agent interacting with other belief systems within a larger-scale complex adaptive system may help explain the unpredictability of outcome in the process of the consultation, as seen through the lens of complexity theory. The consultation is essentially a microcosm of other belief system interactions. In the clinical setting, belief systems influence decisions and ultimately all decision-making is value laden. Evidence-based medicine, so Sackett *et al* say,[48] is 'the integration of best research evidence with clinical expertise and patient values'. So what are these values? Sackett *et al*[49] define them as 'the unique preferences, concerns and expectations each patient brings to a clinical encounter and which must be integrated into clinical decisions if they are to serve the patient.' This seems laudable, if ambitious, but does highlight the fact that patients may have a different mindset to doctors struggling to balance their scientific training with the reality of clinical uncertainty. Taking patients' views into account is good practice, or perhaps a better word in helping the GPR to explore the importance of values would be – care.

Caring and 'love'

One branch of ethics emphasises the caring relationship as a central feature of ethical behaviour (*see* Chapter 10) and perhaps gets close to the relationship many GPs have with their patients.[50] In her relational ethics of care, Noddings[51] sees caring as not simply a matter of feeling favourably disposed towards humankind in general; it requires actual encounters with specific individuals, not merely good intentions. Natural caring is said to exist in us all as children and then, when later distorted by society, it is supplemented by more cognitive ethical caring (tantamount to a virtue) (*see* Chapter 8). This notion of caring comes close to the 'love' described by Maturana and Varela[52] as the 'expression of a biological interpersonal congruence that lets us see the other person and open up for him room for existence beside us'.

In another context, 'love' may also be seen as a binding commitment of agents in a system with one particular aim – even in a military fighting force such as Nelson's fleet at Trafalgar.[53] Often the building of brotherhood through common bonds is enabled by selfless acts such as generosity or sympathy, especially when performed by those perceived to be in a position of power or leadership (such as a doctor). Indeed the emergence of leadership is seen by Griffin as important in linking self-organisation and ethics.[54] He argues that modernist thinking, with its emphasis on the autonomy of the individual, has left us with the notion that 'leaders are quite literally "out" of the ordinary'. Instead, he argues, we should focus on the everyday interactions of people in the living present; ethical behaviour then emerges, as do roles such as leadership or followership. (If you substitute 'doctor' for 'leader' then the parallels become clear.) Griffin characterises ethics as 'a matter of our accountability to each other in our daily relating to each other', adding that 'what is ethical emerges as themes that organise our experience of being together'. He is careful to avoid any statement of principles of ethics that would be context-independent, that is grounded in anything other than the complex responses processes of relating in the living present. In the doctor–patient relationship, an ethical framework will be already forming in a constructive meaning of gestures in a clinical conversation, and that framework will be developed as the conversation continues.[55]

McNamee and Gergen[56] posit the social constructivist view in proposing the ethic of relational responsibility, which culminates in non-linearity and paradox: 'Values sustain community and the community sustains values'.[57] In general practice the reciprocal partnership of community to local GP practice might be seen as similar. There is a responsibility of the practice to serve the community and at the same time the community's participation as patients sustains the nature of the practice. At an individual level, as stated before, the clinician bears a responsibility to the patient to facilitate optimal health and uses a combination of unwritten and written rules or guidance to achieve this end. Clinical guidelines are one such aid, but that is all: they are an aid to a process of moral sensitivity in which the doctor recognises differential values and belief systems must be shared, embraced and acknowledged if optimal health is to be achieved.

Rules which guide behaviour: guidelines

Guidelines may be seen as instructions for action and apply equally to social interaction as medical intervention. Clinical guidelines would be straightforward if simple research showed unambiguously which treatment worked, how low blood pressure should really be, what the best level of cholesterol is. But the world isn't simple and is not predictable. Likewise, ethical behaviour is not always straightforward. So if science and ethical behaviour are uncertain, and evidence constantly changing, how can clinical and ethical decisions be made and what of the role of guidelines? Let's return to our GPR and trainer.

Trainer:	What have you found out about guidelines, with particular reference to the case we discussed yesterday?
GPR:	Well I'm not sure about guidelines. I looked at the NICE and NHS guidelines, and also those from the PCT, and they are all slightly different. Between them they seem to have most of the answers and I tried to follow them but I know that they're not appropriate for every patient.
Trainer:	What you think they are for?
GPR:	I suppose they are to ensure that the best evidence is summarised for doctors and other health professionals to give the best care in practice to their patients.
Trainer:	That seems reasonable, but what about money and resources?
GPR:	Of course that's the job of NICE, isn't it?
Trainer:	Who do you think writes the NICE guidelines?
GPR:	I suppose it's doctors and others ... heavily influenced by government.
Trainer:	Does it matter who writes them?
GPR:	Yes – they need to be user-friendly and relevant locally, but also come from a credible source ...
Trainer:	What about the ethics of guidelines?
GPR:	Well, I suppose they have to achieve different ethical aims, don't they? For example, respecting patient autonomy while fulfilling obligations to use resources well and maximise public health.
Trainer:	So, guidelines are multilayered and have many different purposes?

It is clear that clinical guidelines provide a useful link between what has come to be known as evidence-based medicine and clinical practice. Sackett et al,[58] as we have seen, define evidence-based medicine as 'the integration of best research evidence with clinical expertise and patient values'. However, this begs the question of what one means by, and who defines, 'best research evidence' and 'clinical expertise' as well as the 'patient values' already discussed. Sackett et al's definition, although seen by some as imperfect,[59] is very comprehensive and has been used by governments on both sides of the Atlantic to further the implementation of national guidelines. This, as Goodman points out,[60] can imply that ignorance in an individual clinician can be seen as morally blameworthy.

Ignorance leads to error and error can lead to medical harm. So one view of guidelines might be to reduce error (at an individual level); another might be that they might improve outcomes (at a population level). This mirrors the debate between individual patient and public health, and in ethical terms, a duty-and-rights-based morality versus utilitarianism, well-explored by Rogers, using principle-based ethics as her starting point.[61]

That the use of guidelines is complex is undisputed. The literature on the difficulties in implementing clinical guidelines is growing and the problems of implementation are well-recognised.[62] One problem may be the language of the guideline; for example, simple specific language is often more helpful in changing behaviour than general advice.[63] Language is the key to communication and an important area to consider briefly in considering how the GPR can make an ethical decision using complexity theory to inform her analysis.

Language

Saussure stated that language begins in confusion for words are initially just noises (for the purposes of this chapter, language is assumed to refer to words and oral expression).[64] However, despite the fact that they are arbitrary in origin, words nevertheless communicate information because people have agreed to associate specific sounds with certain relevant parts of the environment. This is a fundamental aspect of all natural processes – what something is and what it means are not the same. For instance, commonly in conversation a new phrase or sentence will arise that has never been said in that particular way or that specific context before, but its meaning is clear to those listening. It is this ability to surprise without confusing that makes language successful and this is accomplished by the fact that to be shared, language must have openly agreed meanings for words and publicly stated grammatical rules for constructing sentences. Language survives and evolves because it sets limits on how we speak without prescribing what we say. Enforcing lower-level activities to follow rules preserves the linguistic system, but liberating expression allows it to evolve to higher levels on which new meanings are constructed and emerge.[65] There is close analogy with other successful evolutionary systems. If the lower-order rules of sentence structure and relationships of words are seen as the interaction of agents in a complex system, then the patterns of meaning that emerge may be seen as the ethical (higher-order) patterns of behaviour that emerge for the system. The simple rules lower down the system generate complex ethical behaviour higher up.

Simple rules

Complexity theory posits the concept of simple rules as a mechanism for explaining the apparently complex behaviour of multi-agent systems. For instance, how do birds flock or fish form shoals? The answer appears in the application of simple local rules. At the first Artificial Life Workshop in 1989, Craig Reynolds demonstrated a computer simulation of bird-flocking behaviour, using three simple rules to dictate the behaviour of his virtual birds or 'boids'. The three rules can be likened to the instructions given to a group of children going on a walk in the park.

1. Keep up (match its own velocity with the boids in its neighbourhood).
2. Don't push (maintain a minimum distance from other objects in the environment, including other boids).
3. Stay together (move towards the perceived centre of the mass of boids).

The emergent pattern of behaviour is both striking and elegant. This demonstrates the patterning and structuring of value sets that occur on a small scale by applying local and not universal rules. The values (and hence ethics) emerge through local iterated interactions. On a larger scale, if we consider a local system to be nested in, and related to, many other local systems, it may be more appropriate to focus on the process by which different contexts can evoke the emergence of such different patterns in the value space, rather than focusing on any particular pattern of values. Context and, specifically, sensitivity to initial conditions is a prerequisite of the emergent behaviour exhibited by a complex adaptive system.[66] Thus, for the GPR, moral sensitivity means more than merely 'moral rela-tivism' – it is a *sine qua non* of establishing and maintaining the fitness of the system within which she and her patient work together to maximise health. Just as a snowflake will vary in shape according to tiny differences in pressure and temperature (while overall apparently conforming to a common hexagonal pattern), so the values that emerge from a local com-plex system will differ according to local rules, history, place, etc. The application of a guideline may have different outcomes when applied by different doctors to different patients in different areas. Like the butterfly effect, consequences can range from the insignificant zephyr to the hurri-cane. The GPR is once again freed: the guideline is not a tyrannical ruler that controls her clinical practice but a tool that will and should be differ-entially used depending on the local complex system within which she is working with patients.

Rules of engagement

The interaction of agents in any system in an ethical way may be seen, as stated, to achieve fitness for the environment. In making decisions though, there is a balance between choosing an action that would benefit only oneself or one that might benefit the larger system at some relative cost to the individual, epitomised by the prisoner's dilemma and now developing into game theory.[67] Agent-based modelling using complexity as an underpinning theoretical concept has shown that rational decision-making using ethical principles often does not tend to occur in a predictable way in complex systems. Many other factors impinge on the decisions made and strategy development is contingent. Linear predictions of outcome are unreliable. Again this resonates clearly with the GPR scenario – the decision was complex and the outcome unexpected, despite the apparent rationality of the guideline-based decision-making process.

At a systems level, if knowing what to do is impossible, then the next best thing is to prepare systems to become adaptable or, in survival terms, to discover threats and generate solutions to them spontaneously. Preserving the capacity of a system to save itself gives substance to an ethics of complexity. Ensuring that the simple rules are the shared values of belief systems – at the grammatical or first-order level – will allow novelty to emerge at the second-order level. In cybernetics terms, the talk would be of second-order control, i.e. rules for rules. Abstracting clinical guidelines to the level of second-order control, rather than specifying first-order actions, may be a useful way for the GPR to think about how clinical guidelines may be best directed.

Learning

Cybernetics is about systematic feedback and learning. At the individual level, a good example for biological learning is that of the immune system, which learns what is self and non-self. Orsucci[68] offers an analogy of bioethics as an immune system:

> In this new perspective, ethical thinking should be considered mostly as a subsystem of the semiotic universe, apt to preserve and maintain the boundaries of the (individual and social) self – a function that is quite similar to the functioning of the immune system: preserving the psychobiological self by discerning what is self, what is non-self; the semiotic agent exploring through confusions and intrusions along fuzzy boundaries. Bioethics works on the edge between body, mind and society just in the same area of functioning of the immune system: in fuzzy and transitional areas between private and public.

Finally the GPR tutorial came to a conclusion.

Trainer:	So what have you learnt about guidelines and ethics?
GPR:	Well, the consultation was difficult because of my interaction with both the patient and the guidelines. Guidelines can be helpful but can be confusing too. I feel my actions and decisions need to be made in partnership with the patient – his views and beliefs must inform my decision. This consultation has also made me think twice about how I might approach discussing BP treatment, both with him and other patients in the future.

The GPR, in interacting with her patient and the guidelines, had become immunised. The exposure to the 'antigens' changed her and in the process she engaged in systemic learning. The same may be said of the patient, but perhaps that remains to be explored in future consultations. In short, the GPR was becoming wiser and more reflective. She would probably act differently in the future and certainly knew a lot more about clinical guidelines!

Conclusion

Medical ethics today is as dynamic as ever and the agenda continues to change as patients and doctors renegotiate their roles.[69] Likewise, complex systems are about adaptation to the environment. As nature evolves novelty arises and one of the novel things that has arisen over the years is ethics. Ethics are no less natural for being created, rather than being deduced and eternal, and no less real for being relative rather than revealing an absolute. While acknowledging the potential criticism of naturalistic fallacy,[70] it is argued that, in viewing clinical interactions as nested complex systems with autonomous agent interaction at a local level, ethical behaviour can be seen as an emergent property of these complex interactions. Emergent ethics as a framework for survival and fitness to the environment means that decisions can be made at the 'razor's edge between moral absolutism and moral relativism'. Reflection on the aim and nature of the system both demands and informs moral sensitivity that is adaptable, applicable and effective. The professional networks of doctors and patients, and the nested and fractal systems of GP surgeries and one-to-one consultations are partially constrained by simple rules. Interpreting these rules and communicating linguistically may bring about novel behaviour and will modify both the local and wider system in the future. The extent of modification is unpredictable, but the emergence of a dynamic clinical ethics of complexity is unavoidable.

It is concluded that:

- insights from complexity offer a novel approach to the study of bioethics and in particular medical ethics: an ethics of complexity linking context with deontological principles through moral sensitivity
- the ethical aspects of guidelines and evidence-based medicine continue to provide a challenge and often cause confusion and anxiety
- complexity theory adds to both the understanding and exploration of ethical implications of guidelines, and also provides a means by which practitioners can feel more confident about the uncertainty, tensions and unpredictability of their work
- in order to become a wise practitioner and to demonstrate moral sensitivity, the health professional must be reflective and adaptable and feel at ease using judgment based on both universal and local rules to guide action in unfamiliar territory.

References

1 Einstein A. Religion and science. *New York Times Magazine*. 9 November; 1930.
2 Grilli R, Lomas J. Evaluating the message: the relationship between compliance rate and the subject of a practice guideline. *Med Care*. 1994; **32**: 202–13; Ellrodt AG *et al*. Measuring and improving physician compliance with clinical practice guidelines (a controlled interventional trial). *Ann Intern Med*. 1995; **122**: 277–82; Conroy M, Shannon W. Clinical guidelines: their implementation in general practice. *BJGP*. 1995; **45**: 371–5.
3 Ferrier BM, Woodward CA, Cohen M, Williams AP. Clinical practice guidelines. New-to-practice family physicians' attitudes. *Can Fam Physician*. 1996; **42**: 463–8.
4 Waldrop M. *Complexity: the emerging science at the edge of chaos*. New York: Simon & Schuster; 1992.
5 Van Uden J, Richardson C, Cilliers P. Postmodernism revisited? Complexity science and the study of organizations. *J Critical Postmodern Organization Science*. 2001; **1**(3): 53–67.
6 Capra F. *The Hidden Connections*. New York: Flamingo; 2003.
7 Mitleton-Kelly E, ed. *Complex Systems and Evolutionary Perspectives on Organisations: the application of complexity theory to organisations*. Oxford: Pergamon Press; 2003.
8 Adapted from Mitleton-Kelly E. *Ibid*.
9 Nicolis G, Prigogine I. *Exploring Complexity*. New York: Freeman; 1989.
10 Arthur BW. *Increasing Returns and Path Dependence in the Economy*. Ann Arbor: University of Michigan Press; 1995.
11 Cilliers P. Knowing complex systems. In: Richardson K, ed. *Managing the Complex: philosophy, theory and applications*. Greenwich, CT: Information Age Publishing; 2004. p. 12.

12 Sweeney K. History of complexity. In: Sweeney K, Griffiths F. *Complexity and Healthcare: an introduction*. Oxford: Radcliffe Medical Press; 2002.

13 Kuhn T. *The Structure of Scientific Revolutions*. Chicago: University of Chicago Press; 1962.

14 Cassirer E, Korner S, Haden J. *Kant's Life and Thought*. New Haven: Yale University Press; 1986.

15 General Medical Council. *Good Medical Practice*. 3rd ed. London: GMC; 2001.

16 De Risio S, Cuomo C. On a possible foundation of ethics. In: De Risio S, Orsucci FF, eds. *Bioethics in Complexity: foundations and evolutions*. London: Imperial College Press; 2004.

17 Atkinson P. Training for certainty. *Soc Sci & Med*. 1984; **19**: 949–56; Atkinson P. *The Clinical Experience: the construction and reconstruction of medical reality*. 2nd ed. Aldershot: Ashgate Publishing; 1997.

18 Neighbour R. *The Inner Apprentice: an awareness-centred approach to vocational training for general practice*. Oxford: Radcliffe Publishing; 2004.

19 Sinclair S. *Making Doctors. An institutional apprenticeship*. Oxford: Berg Press; 1997.

20 Capra F. *The Web of Life*. London: Harper Collins; 1996.

21 Hawking S. *A Brief History of Time*. London: Bantam Press; 1988.

22 Hawking S. *The Universe in a Nutshell*. London: Bantam Press; 2002.

23 Atkinson P. *Medical Work and Medical Talk*. London: Sage; 1995.

24 Millman M. *The Unkindest Cut: life in the backrooms of medicine*. New York: William Morrow; 1976; Cassell J. *Expected Miracles: surgeons at work*. Philadelphia, PA: Temple University Press; 1991.

25 Mol A. *The Body Multiple: ontology in medical practice*. Durham, NC: Duke University Press; 2002.

26 Bosk CL. *All God's Mistakes: genetic counselling in a paediatric hospital*. Chicago: University of Chicago Press; 1995.

27 Strong PM. *The Ceremonial Order of the Clinic*. London: Routledge; 1979.

28 Tallis R. *Hippocratic Oaths: medicine and its discontents*. London: Atlantic Books; 2004.

29 NICE. *Chronic Heart Failure*. http://www.nice.org.uk/pdf/CG5NICEguideline.pdf; 2003 (accessed 29 July 2005).

30 Schön D. *The Reflective Practitioner*. New York: Basic Books; 1983.

31 Berger J. *A Fortunate Man: the story of a country doctor*. New York: Vintage International; 1997.

32 Simon HA. *Models of Bounded Rationality*. Vol 3. Cambridge, MA: MIT Press; 1997; Dowrick C. Uncertainty and responsibility. In: Dowrick C, Frith L, eds. *General Practice and Ethics: uncertainty and responsibility*. London: Routledge; 1999; Goodman K. *Ethics and Evidence-based Medicine*. Cambridge: Cambridge University Press; 2003.

33 *Ibid*. p. 20.

34 Goodman K. *Ethics and Evidence-based Medicine*. Cambridge: Cambridge University Press; 2003. p. 133.

35 Cilliers P. *Ibid*. p. 12.

36 Cilliers P. *Ibid*. p. 17.

37 Smith S. Ethics and postmodernity. In: Dowrick C, Frith L, eds. *General Practice and Ethics: uncertainty and responsibility*. London: Routledge; 1999.

38 Stacey R. *Complex Responsive Processes in Organizations*. London: Routledge; 2001.

39 Kernick D, ed. *Complexity and Healthcare Organisation*. Oxford: Radcliffe Publishing; 2004.

40 Orsucci FF. Ethos in action. In: De Risio S, Orsucci FF, eds. *Bioethics in Complexity: foundations and evolutions*. London: Imperial College Press; 2004.

41 Thompson WI. *Coming into Being: artefacts and texts in the evolution consciousness*. New York: St Martins Press; 1996.

42 Bateson G. *Mind and Nature: a necessary unity*. New York: Dutton; 1979.

43 Maturana HR, Varela FJ. *The Tree of Knowledge*. Boston, MA: Shambhala Publications; 1987.

44 Maturana HR, Varela FJ. *Ibid*. p. 245.

45 Luhmann N. *Social Systems*. Stanford, CA: Stanford University Press; 1995.

46 Teubner G, ed. *Global Law Without a State* (Studies in Modern Law and Policy). Aldershot: Dartmouth; 1997.

47 Maturana HR, Varela FJ. *Ibid*. p. 134.

48 Sackett DL, Straus SE, Richardson WS, Rosenberg W, Haynes RB. *Evidence-based Medicine: how to practice and teach EBM*. Edinburgh: Churchill Livingstone; 2000.

49 Sackett DL *et al*. *Ibid*. p. 1.

50 This is sometimes described as a feminist approach; however, others have distinguished between a feminist and feminine approach to bioethics; *see* Gilligan C. Hearing the difference: theorising connection. *Hypatia*. 1995; **10**(2): 120–7; Held V, ed. *Justice and Care: essential readings in feminist ethics*. Boulder, CO: Westview Press; 1995; Tong R. *Feminist Approach to Bioethics*. Boulder, CO: Westview Press; 1997.

51 Noddings N. *Caring: a feminine approach to ethics and moral education*. Berkeley, CA: University of California Press; 1984.

52 Maturana HR, Varela FJ. *Ibid*. p. 246.

53 Artigiani R. Leadership and uncertainty: complexity and the lessons of history. *Futures*. 2005; **37**: 585–603.

54 Griffin D. *The Emergence of Leadership: linking self organization and ethics*. London: Routledge; 2002.

55 Mishler EG. *The Discourse of Medicine: dialectics of medical interviews*. Norwood, NJ: Ablex Publishing Corporation; 1984.

56 McNamee S, Gergen K. *Relational Responsibility: resources for sustainable dialogue*. Thousand Oaks, CA: Sage; 1999.

57 McNamee S, Gergen K. *Ibid*. p. 20.

58 Sackett DL *et al*. *Ibid*. p. 1.

59 Goodman K. *Ibid*. p. 17.

60 Goodman K. *Ibid*. p. 19.

61 Rogers WA. Are guidelines ethical? Some considerations for general practice. *BJGP*. 2002; **52**: 663–9.

62 Grol R, Grimshaw J. From best evidence to best practice: effective implementation of change in patients' care. *The Lancet*. 2003; **362**: 1225–30.

63 Grol R, Dalhuijsen J, Thomas S, Veld C, Rutten G, Mokkink H. Attributes of clinical guidelines that influence use of guidelines in general practice: observational study. 1998; *BMJ*. **317**(7162): 858–61.

64 Culler J. *Literary Theory: a very short introduction*. Oxford: Oxford University Press; 2000.

65 Artigiani R. *Ibid*. p. 592.

66 Cilliers P. *Complexity and Postmodernism*. London: Routledge; 1998.

67 Axelrod R. *The Complexity of Cooperation*. Princeton: Princeton University Press; 1997.

68 Orsucci FF. *Ibid*. p. 72.

69 *See*, for example, Irvine D. *The Doctor's Tale*. Oxford: Radcliffe Medical Press; 2003; Burke L. Patient loses right-to-food case. BBC News: http://news.bbc.co.uk/2/hi/health/4721061.stm; 2005 (accessed 29 July 2005).

70 Palmer M. *Moral Problems in Medicine: a practical coursebook*. Cambridge: Lutterworth Press; 1999.

Chapter 9

Should doctors observe a moral duty to care for themselves?

Andrew Dicker

> Make the care of your patient your first concern.
>
> General Medical Council, UK

Introduction

The NHS in the UK evolved from one of the most altruistic social policies of the 20th century. There is a prevailing perception that during its several decades of existence it has done a great deal of good for a great many people. But at the beginning of the 21st century there is also a painful understanding of the amount of harm that has paradoxically been caused to people by the NHS in its day-to-day functioning. This harm seems to have been intrinsic to the functioning of the NHS as a provider of socialised medical care funded by taxation. While there must always be an individual context to such things, there is also a collective responsibility for both the good and the harm that has come about as a result of the endeavours of the NHS workforce.

The most overt kind of harm that has occurred, with an apparently continually increasing prevalence, is the harm done to patients. I do not know if the exact amount of harm done to patients has ever been accurately quantified. Doctors are made aware of it mainly through the agency of complaints and litigation. Every NHS provider must have a complaints system, even if no one wants to complain. There is also an undocumented and anecdotal litany of complaints about things which happened to people in their encounters with all parts of the NHS. Every employee of the NHS has been witness to this refrain about the failings of one part or another of the system. The universal availability of systems to deal with complaints does more to promote contempt for the phenomenon of complaining than to deal with its causes and paradoxically diminishes the significance of being complained about.

Complaints may be a reflection of harm perceived to have been done. My concern is about a kind of institutionalised harm about which there is almost never overt complaint or even objection. There is no way to quantify it. The quality of this harm remains covert, but almost every doctor is aware of it. It is the harm done to doctors by doctors themselves. There is a collective denial that harm is either inflicted or felt. This situation is perpetuated by the self-evident truth that doctors, like everyone else, need to look after their physical, mental and emotional wellbeing, but do not. I believe that the harm to which I refer is a consequence of the paternalistic tradition that has been a significant determinant of the professional behaviour of doctors for many decades.

Is paternalism ever acceptable?

Paternalism is deeply embedded in both domestic and workplace culture, and determines much of our day-to-day lives. Most children grow up in families that rely upon paternalistic behaviour to survive. For example, children of an age to have achieved so-called 'Gillick competence' may well consider that it is a good thing to stay in bed until midday and stay up late. Unfortunately, the institutionalised patterns of life, like the hours during which schools function, oblige parents to exercise a degree of paternalism over their otherwise competent children to ensure that they get to school on time. In the workplace, the invasion of managerialism creates a paternalistic environment often resented by the workforce. Paternalism is inescapable in the regulated lives that most of us lead and is often a consequence of institutionalised processes beyond our control. It is only tolerated because it is perceived to be a fundamentally beneficent process.

Immanuel Kant observed that 'paternalism is the greatest despotism imaginable'. Isaiah Berlin, in his essay, *Two Concepts of Liberty*, illuminates Kant's statement further.

> paternalism is despotic, not because it is more oppressive than naked, brutal, unenlightened tyranny, nor merely because it ignores the transcendental reason embodied in me, but because it is an insult to my conception of myself as a human being, determined to make my own life in accordance with my own (not necessarily rational or benevolent) purposes, and, above all, entitled to be recognised as such by others.[1]

The moral requirement for respect for individual autonomy is self-evident in Berlin's analysis.

'Paternalism', in the context of the behaviour of doctors, has become a term to describe a variety of attitudes, learnt behaviour and beneficent intentions that have characterised the relationship between doctor and patient. Implicit in this relationship has been the assumption that the doctor knows better than the patient what is right for the patient. While doctors may possess the knowledge to determine what may be beneficial for particular collective morbidities, it is difficult to understand how doctors can know what the right thing for any individual might be. Despite this tension between the good intentions of doctors and the difficulty of truly respecting the autonomy of the patient in the process, the reason that paternalism has been condemned by generations of authors from Kant onwards is that paternalistic behaviour fails to acknowledge the fundamental importance of the consent of the person for whom the good intentions of the doctor, or anyone else, are intended.

There is a plausible argument that there exist situations in which moderate paternalism is acceptable. This can arise when the need for some benevolent action is so necessary that it should override the requirement for respect for the autonomy of the individual patient and at the same time the need for consent. But this is a relatively rare situation among the millions of encounters between patients and doctors every day in which the principle of necessity does not apply.

The nature of consent

Until very recently the nature of consent has not been properly acknowledged by doctors in general. For consent by anyone to anything to be either meaningful or valid, the person consenting must be fully informed. But if consent can only be valid if the person consenting is *fully* informed about what it is to which they are consenting, then the possibility of valid consent may be an illusion. The state of being fully informed about anything is, after all, very difficult to achieve. To be optimally informed, within the limits of the means of disclosure and understanding, is more realistic and practical. In addition, O'Neill has pointed out that consent should also be rescindable and the amount of information involved should be in the control of the person consenting, in the interest of limiting deception and coercion.[2]

In recent years there has been significant change in the attitude of many doctors towards the fundamental moral importance of attempting to achieve a more valid way of obtaining consent from patients. This is dependent upon emphasis on the need to share understanding between patient and doctor. The effective sharing of understanding is dependent on the skill of the doctor in communicating and the level of trust between patient and doctor.

Most clinicians are familiar with the peremptory request for a patient to sign a consent form indicating consent to a surgical procedure with very little explanation about the procedure itself and uncertainties about its effectiveness, its side effects or alternatives. Many patients will be familiar with the primary care physician who recommends the consumption of anonymous medicines with the advice that their consumption at regular intervals will make the patient feel better. These are two generic examples of paternalistic behaviour by doctors, which probably occur on a daily basis today. Despite the fact that doctors may believe that they are acting in the best interests of their patients, little attention is paid to creating the circumstances in which the consent of the patient can have any validity. In both instances there is an intrinsic assumption that the doctor somehow knows what is right for the patient.

Until very recently, institutionalised paternalism has pervaded the great majority of transactions between patient and doctor. The origins of this despotic culture lie historically in the sources of the professional power of the medical profession. Essentially the professional power of doctors lies in their jealously guarded means of self-regulation and the specialised knowledge that enables them to do their work. The vast and impenetrable literature in which this knowledge has been accumulated has historically only been available to members of the profession. The effects of information technology and globalisation are rapidly undermining this historical power, perhaps to the benefit of everyone.

Because doctors have usually tried to adhere to the moral injunction always to do good, as far as is possible, and, more importantly, to avoid harm, the despotism of professional paternalism has been allowed to continue largely unabated. The general adherence to the ethical principles of beneficence and non-maleficence has perpetuated the notion that the interests of patients must always come first. This principle has invaded the consciousness of doctors and patients alike. Indeed the perpetuation of paternalism has been dependent on the belief that doctors will always put the interests of their patients before their own. This is closely entwined with the acceptance that the doctor knows what is right for the patient.

Putting patients first

The often repeated advice that doctors must always put the interests of their patients first, even before their own interests, has become a kind of *shibboleth* deeply embedded in the professional polemic. It is advice, or sometimes instruction, issued by senior doctors to junior doctors, to encourage them to follow the example set by their senior colleagues. It is an idea recycled by idealistic junior doctors, who perceive lack of commitment among their colleagues or seniors. The same language is used by doctors in general to resist attempts by managers and politicians to impose change in the working practices of doctors. The idea is reciprocally invoked by managers and politicians wishing to impose change in the working practices of doctors, when it becomes a kind of moral blackmail.

In all these contexts it is a harmful *shibboleth* because the underlying message is ambiguous and manipulative. However, it remains a cornerstone of professional paternalism. Because the profession has subscribed to the idea collectively, it has become impossible to resile from it. Indeed, for as long as it continues to be stated, it reinforces the public perception that doctors are on the one hand to be trusted and on the other, should continue to be allowed to know best. This is profoundly hypocritical.

The injunction to put the interests of patients first is hypocritical because it is vacuous, pretentious and impractical. In general, people become doctors because they need to earn a living to pay the mortgage, look after their families, own cars and so on. In the process, doctors may enjoy a rewarding job. Doctors may, in general, wish to do the best they can in the interests of the health of their patients, but they do not in reality put the interests of the patients before their own.

Increasingly, doctors are prone to the growing tensions between their Kantian duty to their individual patients and the imperatives created by centralisation and the associated utilitarian obligations to the wider communities that they serve, often incentivised by financial reward. Perhaps there are a few paragons in the medical community who believe that putting the interests of their patients before their own is the right thing to do. But both in primary and secondary care it has become impossible *literally* to put the interest of patients first because there are too many countervailing forces in the means of delivering ordinary healthcare.

Despite the hypocrisy that underlies the moral imprecation to put the interest of patients first, the advice has been visited and revisited upon successive generations of doctors by doctors. In the paternalistic and hierarchical culture of the medical profession, this erroneous advice has significantly contributed to the reason why doctors have historically failed to look after themselves. This is not exactly the same thing as doctors relegating their own interests to those of their patients. But the failure of doctors to care for themselves is closely related to the institutional behaviour that requires doctors to put the interests of patients before their own.

Institutionalised failure to look after doctors

The professional culture in which medical students and junior doctors in the UK spend their formative years has historically promoted the idea of the selfless doctor working endlessly in the interests of the patients. This culture has been characterised by primitive traditions, which include excessive working hours, lack of peer support, teaching by humiliation, lack of respect for individual needs, sexist attitudes, tribalism, nepotism, bullying,[3] collective denial that anything is wrong, collusion against anyone who tries to change anything and professional suicide for anyone who actively complains or objects about their working conditions.

Most doctors who have trained in the UK will have encountered some or all of these various forms of abuse during their years as a junior doctor working in the secondary care sector. Some will have gone on to senior positions where wittingly or unwittingly they will have revisited the sort of abuse that they encountered during their years in training on the next generation of junior staff. Although the objective evidence for the existence of this cycle of abuse is not available, there is nevertheless a wealth of anecdote on the subject, some of it published.

The problem is not confined to hospital environments. In many apparently harmonious primary care partnerships there prevails a muted tyranny. The paternalistic tradition insidiously invades the relationships between GPs working in partnerships when equity of power within the organisation is not a priority. Even in small organisations, despotic hierarchies emerge where one partner imposes his or her will upon the other partners. Such hierarchies are based on things like length of service, capital shares and workload disparities. Obviously most partnerships function by a consensus of opinion about working practices. But often these work patterns are not established with the willing consent of all concerned but perpetuated by tradition, the deeply held belief of one particular partner or coercion when there is inequity of power within the partnership.

The brutalising effect of these traditional working and learning conditions, all perpetuated in the common cause of putting patients first, has had the paradoxical effect of persuading doctors that it is not acceptable to stop and reflect upon whether their own physical, mental or emotional wellbeing may suffer in the process of their professional development. It is almost unknown for doctors to enquire of each other whether they have been looking after *themselves*.

The need for self-caring doctors

In recent years there have been signs of a cultural change in the climate in which doctors teach and learn. This can be identified by the fashion for promoting life-long learning and the emergence of the reflective practitioner, who is the model doctor embarking on a professional life of learning and practice. It is just possible that part of the reflective process will include some consideration of the doctors' own wellbeing.

Another incentive for the evolution of the self-caring doctor is the tangible increase in defensive practice in the interest of avoiding litigation and complaints. One effect of this change in clinical behaviour is for doctors to ensure that they are actually fit to practice, reinforced by the regulatory organisation and the introduction of appraisal.

In addition to these coercive incentives, there remains a need for a coherent argument to persuade doctors that there is an ethical obligation to look after themselves in order that they remain in the best possible physical, mental and emotional state to provide optimal care for their patients.

The source of such an argument might be found in the consumerist behaviour of patients. Since the 1980s, successive UK governments have promoted the idea that the public should have the right to choice in their selection of services, including healthcare. Consumerist behaviour has been endorsed by politicians as a way of enabling the public to demand what it believes should be provided for general consumption. Consumerist rhetoric has always been framed in the language of rights to give it additional moral authority.

The right to healthcare in the UK, enshrined in legislation, imposes a duty on the Secretary of State for Health to provide the relevant services. This statutory right says nothing about the duty of doctors or anything about how doctors should provide care. It is probably unrealistic to believe that the public should be able to claim a right to be able to consult a doctor who is not only of their choice but who is also up-to-date, well-rested, emotionally stable and physically fit. It would be difficult to substantiate such a claim not least because doctors, like everyone else, are human and prone to exactly the same afflictions as their patients. Imposing such a right, by statute for example, would provide a solution but might be construed as discriminatory. For any kind of right to be meaningful there must exist a correlative duty upon someone else to provide whatever is claimed. To impose a duty on doctors to ensure that they are in the best possible condition to deal with patients would be contentious because it would probably interfere with their individual liberty.

It is doubtful that rights can be proven to exist unless they are created in law or relate to such general and fundamental things as the right to life. This, of course, is a problem when rights are expressed as positive rights, such as a claim to the right for all to universal healthcare.

It is necessary to draw upon the wisdom of Isaiah Berlin once more. Berlin pointed out in his writing on liberty that rights, when expressed negatively, become a much stronger claim than the commonly-heard claim of a right to something expressed in the positive sense. (Rights are discussed in greater detail in Chapter 4.) For example, the proposition that supermarket consumers have a right to be served by a cheerful checkout assistant is a much weaker claim than the possibility that consumers should have a right not to have to be served by a bad-tempered checkout assistant.

In the health market, a reasonable and robust claim might be expressed as the right of the public not to have to consult a doctor who is not fit to fulfil the ordinary duties of a doctor. This is a cogent and plausible claim. It would provide an ethical basis for doctors to fulfil their correlative duty created by the negatively expressed right of the public to access to fit doctors. It would also be the foundation of an ethically framed reason for doctors to look after themselves, something that in the current climate would need to be actively facilitated.

Clearly, in the pursuit of the ethical injunction to avoid harm to their patients, there exists good reason for doctors to look after themselves. It is intimately associated with the requirement to respect the basic right of patients to be self-determining. It is this requirement that has not been sufficiently reflected in the behaviour of doctors towards their patients, allowing the paternalistic tradition of the medical profession to flourish for most of the 20th century and largely ignoring the fundamental, moral importance of the concept of informed consent. Paternalism, and the sort of behaviour that it endorses, has been the source of many of the problems that have afflicted the medical profession in the UK towards the end of the 20th century.

The chronic failure of generations of doctors to look after themselves sufficiently well to ensure that they are fit to look after their patients is arguably a result of not acknowledging that their patients ought to have the right not to have to consult a doctor who is any less than fit to be consulted. This lack of acknowledgement is very similar to the failure of adherence to the ordinary ethical principles that allowed paternalism to become a despotic influence. It starts with a failure of respect for the autonomy of individuals.

The creation of a culture in which doctors observe a duty to look after themselves depends on closer observance, by doctors, of the need to respect the autonomy and right to self-determination both of those whom they would treat as patients and of each other.

It can only be by a shift in the cultural paradigm in which doctors have trained and worked for generations that a serious change could ever occur. It is possible that the progressive feminisation of the medical workforce may be significant as a means of achieving this transition. The male-dominated workforce that characterised the 20th century failed to create a caring profession capable of caring for itself. The predominantly female workforce that, it could be argued, will characterise 21st century primary care may have the capacity to create a more nurturing environment.

It is clearly desirable that doctors should observe a duty to look after themselves, not only because it is a source of benefit to themselves, but because it is a correlative duty to the right the public can reasonably claim not to have to consult unfit doctors. There is a deep sense of paradox that underlies the professional denial that there should be a responsibility for doctors to look after themselves, both individually and collectively. Doctors are, in reality, the best-equipped people to undertake a duty of self-care. After all, it is probably true that accountants look after their own accounts and lawyers, by and large, observe the law. Corporate employees have to undergo the most detailed medical examinations in order to get a job with a big salary and get medical 'check-ups' to retain the right to stay in the corporate pension scheme. Why do doctors ignore their own physical, mental and emotional health?

I have tried to show that there is an ethical imperative that determines that doctors should observe the right of patients to consult doctors who are in an holistically fit condition to be consulted. The practical implication of this is the ironical necessity for the profession to exert its own expert paternalism in a truly beneficent, but wholly consensual way, upon itself by acknowledging that there is a collective need for the healers to pay more attention to healing themselves.

There exists considerable psychological denial that the caring profession need to be cared for. It is deep in the culture, intrinsic to the working lives of doctors, that they must carry on until the job is done, forever 'making the care of the patients their first concern' in unquestioning obedience to the imprecation of their own regulatory body.

The medical profession has always felt a deep sense of insecurity when it is criticised from outside its own ranks. The professional introspection, by means of which doctors judge themselves, is curiously fragile when examined from the lay perspective. This is because doctors seem to have difficulty in looking at their work from any other perspective than a biomedical one, which for them, of course, feels safe. It is only in general practice that there have been serious attempts to examine the process of what actually happens in a consultation between a patient and a doctor. The quality of the experience, for either the patient or the doctor, is a uniquely unmeasurable parameter.

In the context of general practice, the work inspired by Michael Balint has the potential to provide a solution to this problem. At present in the UK, Balint group work is almost completely confined to the educational programmes provided for doctors training to be GPs. In many European countries and in the USA, Balint group work is very widespread and has found a following among a variety of medical specialists, not only GPs and family medicine doctors.

The unique quality of the work of Balint groups is that the method provides a safe environment for doctors to examine the nature of their work with patients from a demedicalised perspective. The members of the group are encouraged to examine the process of the consultation – how the patient came to be in the presence of the doctor; the quality of the relationship between the patient and the doctor; what the patient and doctor felt. The purely biomedical aspects of the case under discussion are deprioritised in order that the emotional quality of the consultation can be revealed.

It may be a relatively simple process to engage doctors in a programme to look after their physical and mental health. The means of addressing the emotional wellbeing of the profession is another rubicon. It is significant that Balint work has been undertaken by only a small minority of GPs over the course of the past 50 years. At the beginning of the 21st century, there are fewer established groups than at any time since Michael Balint started the work. Most hospital doctors have never heard of it and most do not want to. Perhaps the ethical imperative that doctors should take more care of themselves has the potential to change the self-awareness of the profession to a more humanistic approach to its wider needs.

Contained in the title of a well-known book about a Balint group discussing the emotional defences of doctors is a simple and apposite question, which doctors should perhaps ask themselves from time to time: 'What are you feeling, Doctor?'[4] Of course, to answer this question it is first necessary to acknowledge feelings. Historically, doctors have resisted the need to recognise the feelings evoked in the course of their everyday work, sometimes to the point of denial of the existence of feelings altogether. But this, of course, is the greatest emotional defence on which doctors rely and is the cornerstone of professional paternalism.

An earlier version of this chapter was published as a paper in the proceedings of the 13th International Balint Congress held in Berlin in 2003.

References

1 Berlin I. *Two Concepts of Liberty*. Oxford: Oxford University Press; 1969.
2 O'Neill O. Some limits of informed consent. *J Med Ethics*. 2003; **29**(1): 4–7.
3 McAvoy B, Murtagh J. Workplace bullying. *BMJ*. 2003; **326**: 776–7.
4 Salinsky J, Sackin P. *What Are You Feeling, Doctor?* Oxford: Radcliffe Medical Press; 2000.

Chapter 10

Fallible, unlucky or incompetent? Ethico-legal perspectives on clinical competence in primary care

Deborah Bowman

> The bond between a man and his profession is similar to that which ties him to his country; it is just as complex, often ambivalent, and in general it is understood completely only when it is broken: by exile or emigration in the case of one's country, by retirement in the case of a trade or profession.[1]
>
> Primo Levi, *Other People's Trades*

Introduction

In the last decade, the issues of competence, performance[2] and accountability in medicine have taken a significant place on both political and professional agendas, particularly following several high profile cases and public inquiries[3] and the well-publicised responses from the Chief Medical Officer on behalf of the Department of Health.[4] This chapter explores the concept of 'competence' in detail, considering how the ways in which competence is constructed and understood have significant effects on commonly discussed ethico-legal concepts such as duty, accountability and whistle-blowing. In particular, the rhetoric and discourse of professional accountability and self-regulation are analysed with reference to the law and the concepts of duty, consequences and harm, conflicts of interest and trust. I argue that the ways in which professionals identify, understand and define the 'problem' of competence determine the ways in which the core notion of duty is understood and, as such, shapes the ethico-legal response to questions of poor performance, both individually and collectively. A case study is presented and revisited throughout the chapter to elucidate key arguments and principles.

I confine my discussion largely to the concept of clinical competence and the problems of poor performance or under-performance, with particular reference to primary care. Many readers will be aware that there is a voluminous and growing literature on medical error and patient safety. While error and mistakes frequently lead to concerns about a clinician's performance, and there are potential implications for patient safety when a healthcare professional under-performs, the broader topics of clinical error and patient safety are not the focus of this chapter. Instead, I discuss the situation where a pattern of behaviour and performance (which may indeed involve error and raise concerns about patient safety) has emerged over time, such as to raise questions about the professional's competence,[5] and discuss the ways in which colleagues and other professionals may respond to those questions. Finally, the focus of this chapter is largely medical. However, I hope that the principles described, and the discussion thereof, are sufficiently well-elucidated to make the chapter of interest to the range of professionals who work in healthcare in general and primary care in particular.

Deconstructing and constructing competence

This section describes the formal or external mechanisms by which a doctor's competence and standards of performance can be defined and reviewed, i.e. the institutions, systems and processes by which standards are defined and performance is reviewed and, if appropriate, sanctioned. I have identified three sources that shape the formal representation of what it means to be a competent doctor, namely:

• the law
• professional bodies
• policy.

Although each category is discussed separately, there is frequently overlap and interaction between the categories; for example, a doctor may be both a defendant in a negligence action and the subject of the General Medical Council's (GMC) fitness to practise procedures. Further, the overlap is illustrated by the fact that professional bodies are established by, and work within, a legal framework and that in order to implement policy, legislation is required and case law will often follow. This section should therefore be read with this overlap in mind.

The law

The law provides the framework within which the medical profession regulates itself, the principal statutes being The Medical Acts 1858 and 1983 (as amended).[6] The GMC has been in existence for nearly 150 years.[7]

The GMC currently has four functions, namely to maintain the register of medical practitioners,[8] provide ethical guidance to inform the work of doctors,[9] inform and quality-assure medical education and training[10] and conduct fitness-to-practise procedures.[11] In 2003, the Council for Healthcare Regulatory Excellence (CHRE) was established[12] as an over-arching body with the power to review the regulatory function not just of the GMC, but of all nine healthcare regulatory organisations. The CHRE has discretion under s 29(1) of the National Health Service Reform and Healthcare Professions Act 2002 to refer decisions of the GMC's fitness-to-practise panels to the High Court if those decisions are believed to be unduly lenient.[13]

Recent years and, at the time of writing, even recent weeks, have seen considerable challenge to the GMC. Following much discussion and high-profile expressions of disappointment about the GMC's rate of progress in advancing the recommendations of public inquiries,[14] the Chief Medical Officer published two consultation papers proposing radical reform of medical and healthcare regulation in July 2006. The consultation paper on medical regulation contains far-reaching proposals, and reveals a transformed socio-political landscape. In short, the consultation paper challenges the essence of self-regulation. The consultation paper makes proposals in respect of fitness to practise, revalidation and 'relicensing', local supervision of doctors and undergraduate medical education. If the proposals become law, the GMC will see a significant diminution in its powers. Of the four regulatory responsibilities previously fulfilled by the GMC, two would be transferred to other organisations, one would be shared with another body, leaving only one remaining.

What are the details of these proposals[15] that have already caused considerable disquiet amongst the profession? First, the GMC's adjudicatory power in fitness to practise cases will transfer to a new tribunal, thereby separating the investigative and adjudicative functions of regulation. The burden of proof will be lowered to the civil from the criminal standard in conduct, health and performance cases. A network of 580 practising doctors paired with a lay person will act as 'affiliates' in each NHS Trust to record and convey local 'concerns' about doctors to be collated and retained centrally. Revalidation will be required every five years and relicensing will depend on a 'strengthened' system of appraisal against benchmark standards based on a contractual 'good doctor' blue print. The blue print would be determined by the GMC, but in conjunction with patient groups and the Postgraduate Medical Education and Training Board. Thus, the second of the GMC's four functions is compromised and the freedom to set standards will no longer reside exclusively with the Council. As well as revalidation, doctors will be required to undergo specialty-specific 'recertification' for which their practice will be evaluated against standards set by the relevant Royal College. Finally the GMC's responsibility for undergraduate medical education will transfer to the Postgraduate Medical Education and Training Board, thereby removing the second of the GMC's four functions. The consultation period ended on 10 November 2006, and for now, the statutory framework remains largely unaltered from the time the GMC was established, but 2006 was unquestionably a time of significant change in medical regulation.

In relation to the work of healthcare professionals, section 18(1) of the Health Act 1999 imposes a duty of quality on all those working in the NHS. It is this provision that underpins the principles of clinical governance:[16] the formalisation of a professional duty to scrutinise practice with the aim of maintaining and improving standards in the broadest sense.[17] Clinicians have a collective responsibility, therefore, not only to reflect on their own practice but also to be aware of and, if necessary, respond to the practice of colleagues even in the absence of formal line-management responsibilities. Further important policy developments under the Health Act 1999 are described below.

A third statute that may be relevant to those concerned with a doctor's performance is the Public Interest Disclosure Act 1998, which provides protection for those who express formal concern about a colleague's performance. The expression of concern must constitute a 'qualifying disclosure', be expressed using appropriate procedures and be made in good faith. An important provision of the Act in relation to GPs is that its terms apply to workers and not just 'employees'; therefore the independent contractor status of many GPs does not preclude them from protection under the 1998 Act. While the law clearly seeks to support those who make the difficult decision to blow the whistle, its effect in practice may be limited. Although 'disadvantage' and 'dismissal' are prohibited by the Act, it cannot prevent intense discomfort, isolation and subtle expressions of hostility.[18]

The law of torts, in particular negligence case law, is another source of what standards of care might be expected of a competent doctor. A test established in the case of *Bolam v Friern Management Committee*[19] provided the basis for defining the standards against which a doctor's actions are judged. The test asks whether a defendant's actions fall short of those of a body of reasonable practitioners (which need not be the *majority* of practitioners). Therefore, on the application of the *Bolam* test, if an expert witness stated that a doctor's actions were those of a reasonable practitioner, it was most unlikely that he or she would be found negligent. The

Bolam test was criticised by those who believed that it invested the power to make determinative judgment in medical opinion (as represented by medically qualified expert witnesses).[20] The test was also perceived as flawed because it equated commonly accepted practice with acceptable practice.[21]

In 1997, the House of Lords held in *Bolitho v City and Hackney Health Authority*[22] that the court was not bound to accept that a doctor had not been negligent merely because expert opinion affirmed that a defendant's actions accorded with those of a reasonable body of his peers. The House stated that, in order to be judged 'reasonable', a defendant's actions (and the expert's opinion of those actions) should be capable of withstanding logical analysis by the court. Thus, for the first time, there was a clear statement by the most senior members of the judiciary that courts should scrutinise medical opinion rather than simply accept the assessments of expert witnesses.

The decision generated much comment in both the professional and academic medico-legal press, and was interpreted (and indeed welcomed) by many as marking the demise of the power of the medical profession to determine an appropriate standard of care.[23] However, in practice, I would argue that it is likely that only a negligible number of cases will produce expert opinions that are so unreasonable that they do not withstand logical analysis.[24] Furthermore, as McHale points out, 'their Lordships were, in fact, quite circumspect in their approach'.[25] It would seem that although in theory the perceived protection afforded to the medical profession by the *Bolam* test has been modified by the judgment in *Bolitho*, in practice the effect of such a modification is likely to be limited and perhaps the real power of the decision is, as McHale goes on to suggest, in sending out a signal for future clinical litigation.[26]

Aside from the interpretative character of the standard of care tests used in court, there are further limits to using the law of negligence as a definitive source for defining the competent practitioner. First, case law is a partial and skewed corpus of material: many of the most catastrophic cases of clinical negligence never reach the court and are therefore never subject to, nor contribute to the evolution of, the legal standard of care because they are settled out of court (i.e. a payment is made on behalf of the defendant doctor or health authority to the claimant before the case is heard in court).

Secondly, for a claim of negligence to be instigated, not only must the patient have suffered damage, but he or she must have sufficient insight to question whether the care provided by the doctor may have fallen below the appropriate standard of care. This is no mean feat for a non-expert. One of the reasons that *Bolam* remained the accepted test of the standard of care in clinical negligence for so long was because the courts necessarily relied on medical expertise because the ability of non-clinicians to understand, still less assess, the quality of medical care provided is often limited. If the powerful and disinterested legal system struggles to evaluate medical care, it is even more difficult for a patient.

Even if a patient does question the standard of the medical care received, there are other variables that influence whether a patient instigates a legal claim.[27] Indeed, in respect of primary care, the doctor–patient relationship has been cited as a legal prophylaxis because GPs have a more personal relationship with their patients; therefore errors and poor outcomes are more likely to be forgiven than in the comparatively impersonal environment of secondary care.[28] Furthermore, negligence actions are expensive and many patients simply do not have the financial resources to bring a claim.

Finally, and perhaps most fundamentally, the equation of competence and negligence is, it is submitted, ultimately unhelpful. Given the fallibility of human endeavour, any doctor may make an error that constitutes negligence. However, this does not render that doctor incompetent. It is generally accepted that inherent in the definition of incompetence is time, i.e. *patterns* of error or *repeated* failure to learn from error.[29] In short, many doctors who have been held to be negligent are competent and many incompetent doctors will never have been, nor will be, held to be negligent.

Professional bodies

Professional bodies such as the GMC, British Medical Association (BMA) and the Royal Colleges have diverse but often overlapping roles in developing, defining and revising standards for doctors.[30] The general remit of the GMC has been described. Now it is worth examining the specific guidance provided by the GMC in greater detail, specifically in relation to the issues of competence and under-performance.

The principal publications in which the GMC sets out standards and obligations relating to competence and performance are *Duties of a Doctor* and *Good Medical Practice* (currently under review).[31] *Duties of a Doctor* sets out 14 broad principles, each of which could be said to contribute to defining the competent doctor, but three are of particular relevance, as listed here.

- Keep his or her professional knowledge and skills up to date.
- Recognise the limits of his or her professional competence.
- Act quickly to protect patients from risk where he or she has good reason to believe that a colleague may not be fit to practise.

Good Medical Practice is a much more detailed document and states that a doctor must perform satisfactorily in a range of domains:

- providing competent clinical care
- maintaining the standards of his or her practice over the course of his or her career
- providing fair and accurate references and assessments and fulfilling teaching and training responsibilities
- developing and maintaining good relationships with patients
- having effective and functional relationships with colleagues
- acting with probity
- considering the implications of his or her health for medical work.

Good Medical Practice provided the basis for the RCGP (in collaboration with the GMC's General Practitioners' Committee) to publish guidance on what standards are required of GPs.[32] *Good Medical Practice for General Practitioners* adds considerably to the broad domains of *Good Medical Practice*. It not merely enunciates standards of care, however, but also offers descriptors by which a GP's practice can be judged to be excellent or unacceptable. It is a comprehensive starting point for anyone seeking guidance on competence in general practice, notwithstanding the somewhat curiously binary choice of assessing a professional's work as either aspirant 'excellence' or depressing 'unacceptability'.

The RCGP has also published much supporting documentation on quality[33] and revalidation,[34] and guidance for professionals who have concerns about a GP's performance.[35] However, as will be discussed later in the chapter, the proliferation of high-quality information does not necessarily make the resolution of individual cases straightforward.

Policy

Since Labour came to power and published the *NHS Plan*,[36] there has been an exponential number of policy reforms shaping the ways in which the medical competence and accountability agenda have evolved. For example, there are now far more organisations concerned broadly with quality and performance in the NHS. Even the government expressed concern about the multiplicity of organisations and, in October 2003, instigated a review of 'arm's-length bodies' with a view to reducing the number from 38 to 20.[37] This seemed to be acknowledgement that too many organisations, producing an excess of documents, duplicating effort and jostling for position in the consciousness of busy staff could damage rather than enhance standards of care across the NHS.

The increased scrutiny of doctors' competence found further policy translation in the prominence of appraisal and revalidation, as already discussed. There have been other policy initiatives that adopted the rhetoric of quality, such as increased use of clinical and administrative targets, PFI initiatives and the development of specialist screening facilities and treatment centres, assessment of performance by NHS trusts and the expansion of medical education and training. Detailed discussion of these myriad initiatives is beyond the scope of this chapter, but interested readers could do no better than to consult the thought-provoking critique offered by Pollock.[38]

Given the range of sources available to those seeking external guidance on competence and performance in medicine, and in particular in general practice, why do performance problems remain among the most challenging of all ethical dilemmas? The clue may be the word 'ethical'. Pellegrino and Thomasma[39] argue that the inherent humanity of the doctor and the patient endows the clinical encounter with a moral force that is more powerful than basic legal rules, guidelines and codes of conduct. Medicine, for Pelligrino and Thomasma, is part science, part art and part virtue (*see* Toon in Chapter 6). Jacob,[40] commenting on Pelligrino and Thomasma, also accepts that ethics have regulatory function. Jacob frames regulation as something to which the medical profession reacts. However, given the determination with which the profession has fought (and may continue to fight) to protect the principle of self-regulation, it could equally be argued that the profession is proactive not reactive and shapes the nature of its own regulation. Regulation may be necessary but it will rarely be sufficient. As such, the place of ethical analysis is integral to the identification and management of a performance problem – and ethical analysis is difficult.

The construct of competence: knocking it down and building it up

The naming of a problem is not a neutral process. Implicit in the identification, interpretation and presentation of a problem are values, preferences and choices, which may reflect deeper philosophical and political allegiances. For example, what a patient values may be quite different from what the doctor values and this difference may result in disparity in how each party defines competence. The place of values is particularly evident when reviewing the ways in which clinical competence has been considered by academics and professionals, even without taking into account patient perceptions.[41] The literature on clinical competence reveals writers who have focused variously on systems,[42] individual responsibility and personal experience,[43] the taxonomy and classification of error,[44] intention and the moral aims of doctors and medicine,[45] quantitative measures of performance and statistical analyses of outcomes,[46] stress, ill-health, psychology and other influences on competence,[47] professional identity, power and collective culture,[48] and responses to errors or poor performance.[49] These differences are important. They are not just indicative of vital academic debate, but demonstrate first, how difficult it is merely to name the problem with which one is dealing when reflecting on clinical performance, and second, how the ways in which one eventually elects to name the problem determine ensuing analysis and decisions.

In naming the problem of competence, which components might be deconstructed and analysed? Knowledge appears to be the easiest element of competence to assess, but knowledge itself is not a neutral concept, either in content or in function. Indeed, the development and uses of biomedical knowledge have long been a rich topic for philosophers, sociologists and anthropologists. Why does it matter how knowledge is understood? Knowledge and its contribution to medical work matters because it shapes how competence is understood. A reductionist approach to medical knowledge in which biomedicine is characterised as scientific, coherent and consistent[50] means competence is measurable only against the known. However, if biomedical reductionism exists alongside humanist and holistic models, the definition of competence broadens so that judgments about the practice of another GP may become easy to avoid. The knowledge base of general practice could allow GPs simultaneously to defend a preferred definition of competence while acknowledging that there are competing definitions, thereby absolving doctors of the obligation to judge the competence of others, yet preventing outsiders from legitimately assessing performance. This may partially explain why a participant in Rosenthal's study on poorly performing doctors believed that 'the consultants are a tea party to engage, compared to the GPs'.[51]

Since the 19th century, medicine has been presented as having a positivist scientific knowledge base. The current emphasis on evidence-based medicine serves to reinforce the importance of the knowledge in medicine. (For further discussion of evidence in general practice, *see* Chapter 6.) As challenges to the applicability of evidence-based medicine have gathered momentum, the profession, particularly in primary care, has explored other bases for their work. Recently, narrative-based medicine has become influential in professional and academic analyses of medical work[52] and increasingly the humanities are part of medical training. Since Kuhn[53] asked a chemist and a physicist whether an atom of helium was a molecule and elucidated multiple realities and the concept of the paradigm in science, claims to value-free and culturally-neutral knowledge have been questionable and questioned.

Readers may feel impatient with the intellectual nihilism of social constructionism when considering biomedicine with its incontrovertible truths derived from fundamental principles of physiology, pathology and anatomy. Perhaps, however, the truths are rarer than the dynamic, complex, messy, non-linear uncertainties that constitute much of medicine. And, just as Kuhn tackled the 'hard' sciences by asking an apparently simple question, so in biomedicine, philosophers and social theorists have considered medical pathologies and tasks that could be considered to be at the core of positivist medical knowledge and truths. Two examples are Mol's absorbing ethnography of the ways in which atherosclerosis is defined, represented, explained, measured, managed and reinterpreted to produce a cohesive account in a Dutch hospital[54] and Atkinson's study of a haematology team and the ways in which imaging, microscopy, investigations and clinical meetings contribute to the construction and reconstruction of medical events (including errors).[55] Even if one rejects the idea that scientific knowledge is socially constructed and culturally located, the relevance of 'pure' biomedical knowledge in primary care as a means of determining competence may be questionable. The nature of primary care means that 'pure' scientific knowledge has to be shared with, for example, communication skills, advocacy, psychology, familiarity with support networks and the management of time, resources and personnel.

It is not only the ways in which knowledge is constructed, represented and changes that is relevant to the issue of competence. The functions and uses of biomedical knowledge also have implications for an analysis of what it means to be competent and, more importantly, who should decide who is competent. Since the early 1950s, academics, many of whom were sociologists, have been considering the extent to which knowledge bestows power on those who have medical expertise. In a seminal paper, Hughes[56] argued that in response to mistakes, a profession will build defences against the outside world. An important part of these defences is to establish devices that allow members of the profession to define what constitutes a mistake and what methods should be adopted to address mistakes. If one develops this thesis to its logical conclusion, it is not merely in the case of mistakes that another medical colleague may arguably be seen to be best equipped to name it as an error, but also in relation to judging the much more fundamental concept of professional competence.

Later, Foucault[57] developed a distinct theory of power in his explorations of medical knowledge and the medical profession. He was not concerned solely with the professionalisation of medical practice (unlike the sociologists): his theoretical focus was much broader, more dispersed and uniquely challenging. Foucault refused to hang his theories and arguments about the nature of medical practice on a single concept. Thus, it was neither the professional identity of doctors, nor the scientific revolution and demise of religion, that defined the medical profession. Foucault did not focus on any single area of medical action: he was as concerned with the dyadic encounter as the effect of disease on large populations. He argued that power and knowledge in medicine are subtle, dispersed, sometimes chaotic, non-linear and multi-factorial, thereby revealing the diverse nature of medical practice. This is important because once the diverse nature of medical practice is revealed, then so too is the diverse and amorphous nature of competence in medicine.

Foucault's analysis has been criticised because it disregards the moral aspects of medical work and practice. Good comments that Foucault's omission of morality is significant because 'it is precisely the conjoining of the physiological and soteriological that is central to medicine as a modern institution'.[58] The use of the word 'soteriological' is fascinating. Could it be that to describe medicine as work incorporating salvation or deliverance is to reveal that, notwithstanding the rise and rise of biomedicine, notions of spirituality and religious mysticism remain important to the practice of medicine? Whether morality is an inherent part of medical work *per se*, or related to the standard of care offered by individual doctors continues to be debated in the ethical literature.[59]

Any discussion of clinical competence must address uncertainty. Fox[60] has argued that uncertainty is inevitable and falls into two categories. The first refers to the limitations of an individual doctor's knowledge; the second (and more significant) describes the intrinsically limited nature of medical knowledge itself. Medicine is incomplete, controversial and contested, and there remains an infinite amount of unanswered, and perhaps unanswerable, questions. It is, posits Fox, the conflation of these two types of uncertainty with which every doctor must learn to cope in medical practice. In the context of primary care, uncertainty has been the subject of much analysis and discussion.[61] Leaders of the profession have suggested that uncertainty is characteristic of general practice – the 'risk sink' of medicine.[62] Add inherent uncertainty to the mix of contested knowledge, skills and behaviours required in general practice and the quest for a clear understanding of competence becomes yet more complex.

Do the complexity and diverse perceptions of competence that I have presented lead to a perpetual cycle of infinite deconstruction and ultimate paralysis when grappling with the problem of poor performance?

I do not believe so. Rather, the purpose of exploring, even to a limited extent, the contested and various ways in which competence can be understood is to argue for the importance of naming the problem in ethical analysis and demonstrating that there are multiple ways in which the problem can be understood. If concern is expressed about a doctor, the first ethical duty of his colleagues is to explore the diverse perspectives of those involved and negotiate the naming of the problem. It is only by this process that an appropriate response can be provided – values, interpretations, perceptions and opinions are not irritants to be neutralised in the pursuit of an illusory objective process, but integral to providing a fair and transparent process.

From theory to practice

The case of Dr M

Dr M has been working as a partner in a GP practice for a year, having moving to the area from a city 300 miles away. He has been a GP principal for 12 years and came highly recommended by his last practice.

Since his appointment, Dr M has become increasingly unreliable and disorganised in his work. He has often turned up late for surgeries, neglected to return telephone calls, mislaid correspondence and missed practice meetings at which he was expected to participate in significant event analyses of cases in which he was involved. Two of Dr M's partners have separately told the senior partner of occasions when Dr M appeared not to have performed an appropriate examination on patients, and when he has made 'odd' prescribing and management decisions. At an educational meeting, two local consultants expressed concern 'informally' to the senior partner about Dr M's management of patients and the quality of his referral letters. While Dr M is on annual leave, a locum approaches the senior partner to express 'grave concern' about Dr M's performance. The locum has, in the short time he has been covering for Dr M, found a number of examples where he believes Dr M has 'put patients at risk'.

Pulled in all directions: conflicts of interest

For those who are concerned about a doctor's performance, there will be conflicts of interest. Ethically, conflicts of interests are important because they influence and sometimes determine the ways in which we perceive and respond to a problem.[63] Traditionally, in the ethico-legal literature, conflicts of interest have been characterised as denoting personal or professional gain, often in a financial sense.[64] However, as in my preceding discussion on knowledge and competence, there are more subtle ways in which conflicts of interest can and should be considered. Consulting styles, prescribing choices and preferences for particular consultants are all likely to influence a GP's practice. If a fellow GP doesn't share these preferences, how might this affect a judgment of competence? It is relatively easy to recognise a financial or political conflict of interest, but it is more difficult to recognise these subtle, yet potentially powerful, influences on how one constructs general practice and therefore the competent practitioner.

So, after naming the problem, the second stage in the ethical process is to consider conflicts of interest, as widely as possible. I once worked with a GP who had been taught in medical school that, wherever possible, he should not prescribe more than three drugs per patient otherwise iatrogenic effects would ensue. What might the implications be for this GP's colleagues who may be more comfortable with polypharmacy? Is this merely a pharmacological philosophical difference or a matter of competence? More importantly, would this difference ever come to light unless it were first identified as a difference and discussed?

In the case of Dr M, potential conflicts of interest abound. First, the senior partner is likely to feel loyalty towards Dr M as a close colleague, and perhaps even a friend. It may be significant that it is an outsider, i.e. the locum, who has raised concerns about Dr M's performance. It has been argued that those who raise concerns about clinical performance are, like the locum in the case study, most likely to be new to existing organisations and systems.[65] The ties that bind GPs in partnership are considerable and perhaps more fundamental than is routinely acknowledged. Discussing how doctors in different specialties perceive and experience stress, Firth-Cozens notes that of 124 GPs who participated in her study, only four did not have siblings.[66] Firth-Cozens hypothesises that, 'It may be that they [the GPs in the study] went into this "working family" of partnership in order to recapture or make good their early family experiences.'[67] Whether one accepts this psychoanalytical approach to understanding why and how GPs work in groups, it is extremely difficult for those in a partnership to address concerns about performance and this difficulty is often felt more acutely in primary than in secondary care.[68]

In addition to the personal loyalty to Dr M as a colleague, there may be financial conflicts of interest. Surgeries are small businesses and the impact of disrupting the partnership is considerable. The impact of dissolving partnership is even greater. Inevitably these factors, while perhaps not vocalised, will have a bearing on how the senior partner perceives and responds to the locum's concerns. In addition to the inconvenience and cost of losing Dr M's services either temporarily or permanently, there may be less quantifiable effects on the reputation of the practice, the relationship of the practice with external parties who may have an interest in Dr M's performance, for example the primary care trust, the ways in which Dr M's difficulties reflect on those who appointed him as a partner and staff workload.

It is to be hoped that Dr M isn't also a patient of the practice where he is a partner,[69] but he may be, given that significant numbers of doctors don't register with a GP,[70] self-medicate,[71] or find seeking help difficult.[72] The senior partner might ensure that Dr M has access to advice and support outside the practice, for example, a GP, support organisations[73] or an occupational health service. For detailed discussion on whether there is an ethical imperative to self-care, *see* Chapter 9.

Duty and consequences

Having argued that naming the problem and considering conflicts of interest broadly are the first two stages in responding ethically to the locum's concerns, this section explores the ways in which core ethical concepts of duty and consequences further inform the analysis – an exercise in applied ethics. In brief, the concepts of duty and consequences are derived from two important moral theories, namely deontology and consequentialism. Deontology proposes that morality is determined by principles that should be followed irrespective of consequences; it is a theory in which principle denotes intrinsic morality. In the case of Dr M, one might ask whether there are principles or obligations that are relevant to the case, for example, with regard to truth-telling, putting patients first above all other groups or respect for persons. Consequentialism, in contrast, seeks to explore problems with reference to the likely consequences: in the case of Dr M, one might ask what the consequences of possible actions or inactions might be. For example, are there circumstances in which truth is likely to have adverse consequences for Dr M himself or patients? What would the net gains and losses be if the practice suspends or even dismisses Dr M? How would decisions affect Dr M's career and wellbeing?

Although there is a clear difference between deontology and consequentialism, it may be misleading to imply that a theoretical choice has to be made. The development of moral obligations and rules is often informed by likely consequences. It is also possible simultaneously to make deontological and consequentialist points to support a moral position. For example, consider this quotation from Ken Livingstone, writing about the moral choices facing Britain following terrorist attacks in London.

> Those believing he [Qaradawi] should be banned give lip service to treating Britain's Muslim community with respect but in practice deny it. Not only is that wrong itself, but it will increase the number of alienated fanatics.[74]

The case of Dr M and the question of duty

The work of the GMC in regulating the profession does not reach the majority of practising doctors.[75] Even though there have been suggestions recently that the GMC is being over-zealous in pursuing doctors about whom there are concerns,[76] it remains likely that expressions of concern will be shared, initially and perhaps exclusively, with other clinicians and possibly managers. The discretion of first-line responders is considerable and the ways in which those initially approached, such as the senior partner in the case study, choose to interpret the problem and subsequently respond carries considerable moral and professional responsibility.

The senior partner and Dr M's other colleagues may feel that they owe duties to two parties, namely patients and Dr M himself. Using Dworkin's[77] terminology, the duty to patients is clear, 'trumps' the duties to Dr M and the profession, and is reinforced by the GMC, which states unequivocally 'you must make the care of the patient your first concern' and:

> you must protect patients from risk of harm posed by another doctor's ... conduct, performance or health[78] ... the safety of patients must come first at all times. Where there are serious concerns about a colleague's performance, health or conduct, it is essential that steps are taken without delay to investigate the concerns to establish whether they are well-founded, and to protect patients.[79]

These ethical imperatives could be said to be based on the principle of respect for persons. Patients are not means to an income, professional security or self-worth, but ends in themselves. Patients are dependent upon doctors for care and they do not come to the relationship with equal status or knowledge. Put simply, most patients trust their doctors: they believe they are competent. Thus Dr M's colleagues have a duty to investigate the locum's concerns and consider these concerns in the context of the behaviours other partners have observed. The only way in which the ethical imperative to place patients first can be fulfilled is to address the concerns about Dr M's performance.

If, as seems likely, there is reason to be concerned about Dr M's competence, it is likely that the senior partner will want to talk to Dr M directly. In the course of this conversation, it is possible for the senior partner to have regard to the secondary duty of care to Dr M himself by offering advice and support, provided that the senior partner does not lose sight of his primary duty – to protect patients. If Dr M accepts that there are problems with his performance, it may be possible to negotiate actions that will ameliorate the situation, particularly if careful and close attention is played to naming the problem and matching the response. For instance, is the problem a knowledge deficit (educational remediation, mentoring and perhaps supervised practice may be appropriate), is it a health or stress-related problem (access to independent support, advice and treatment are indicated) or are there systems problems (attention to the surgery and its ways of working would be warranted)?

If, as is perhaps more likely, Dr M does not accept there is a problem with his performance, how should the senior partner proceed? Again, the GMC is clear:

> You must give an honest explanation of your concerns to an appropriate person from the employing authority ... If there are no appropriate local systems, or local systems cannot resolve the problem, and you remain concerned about the safety of patients, you should inform the relevant regulatory body.[31]

It is likely that the next stage for the senior partner would be to contact the clinical governance lead at the primary care trust. Another source of advice is the National Clinical Assessment Service (formerly the National Clinical Assessment Authority),[80] which draws on its national and international expertise in performance problems while emphasising local resolution. Although the senior partner is ethically obliged to act, concerns have been established about Dr M's performance, the emotional impact of discharging this obligation is considerable and there is notable ambivalence about the role of whistle-blowers, beautifully encapsulated by Hunt, who describes those who blow the whistle as 'a peculiar and fascinating hybrid ... half trouble-maker, half-hero'.[81] The senior partner may wish to identify a trusted mentor or third party with whom he can debrief.

Consequentialism and the relevance of harm

If there is, as I have argued, an ethical obligation to tackle the question of Dr M's performance once the concerns are found to be warranted, is there any place for a consequentialist analysis of the problem? Reviewing the source of the principle that demands action by the senior partner and the broader literature on performance and accountability in medicine, it is evident that consequences are very important. The GMC invokes the concept of risk repeatedly in its statements that doctors must act in the event of poor performance. Clearly medicine is a risky enterprise, but the moral acceptability of risk is connected to competence. Thus most would accept that a surgeon conducting an operation may have 70% mortality rate, provided he has done all he can to ensure he is proficient at performing the operation, that he performs it to the best of his ability and that he reviews his practice to ensure that he remains acceptably proficient; but not if the same surgeon has a 70% mortality rate for an operation for which he is inadequately trained, that he conducts with a hangover or other impairment and that he chalks up to experience. Doctors must put themselves in the best position to be competent notwithstanding the inherent risks of medicine: the moral difference is between avoidable and unavoidable mistakes.[82]

Implicit in the emphasis on consequences is harm, which prompts the question of whether poor performance matters independent of consequences. It is submitted that poor performance matters very much whether or not harm is likely or ensues: patients come to doctors expecting a basic level of competence and care, and the relationship depends on trust. A surgery makes representations to patients that foster and maintain trust. Representations that a doctor is someone in whom a patient should place his trust inform the whole process of seeking care – from a plaque on the wall bearing a doctor's name, credentials and status to offering appointments with, and providing a consulting room for, individual doctors. If Dr M continues to practise at the surgery while there are serious concerns about his performance, this is ethically unacceptable, irrespective of the risk of harm, because it indicates collective misrepresentation and dishonesty by the practice.

Moving on: responses to poor performance

Finally, is there an ethical way in which to move on from performance problems? The literature suggests that there is a moral imperative to learn both individually and collectively from medical error if not poor performance. In a fascinating review of error reporting in the nascent specialty of neurosurgery between 1890 and 1930, Pinkus demonstrates how the focus on positive results in medicine was not always the preferred model.[83] Indeed, just as medical research shapes and limits not only the knowledge base but also the culture and identity of medicine, so too does professional and academic publishing. Could it be that there is an ethical imperative, if not to publish, at least to share experiences of assessing and responding to performance problems? May we yet see the day when *The International Journal of Medical Errors, Poor Performance and Negative Findings* takes pride of place on journal subscription lists?

Certainly, there has been a long-held view that there is an imperative to learn from error, if not more generalised patterns of poor performance. Charles Bosk's work[84] describes how young surgeons are expected to respond to their errors by remembering and learning. The value and desirability of learning is evident in the importance attributed to significant event and critical incident analyses where participation is now a professional obligation. If there is a moral obligation to learn from discrete events and individual clinical cases, could this be part of a wider imperative to review how one assesses and responds not only to one's own performance, but also to that of colleagues?

Conclusions

The issue of accountability in medicine remains topical: media sensationalism, public perception, the medical profession's (sometimes justified) frustration at the avaricious and mercenary lawyer swooping on errors, and the legacy of a belief that to criticise one's colleagues is simply inappropriate, have all contributed to a situation where the key players have taken up sometimes intractable and often poorly-reasoned positions in the debate. In this chapter, I have argued that a rigorous and ethical response to performance problems in healthcare demands that the participants engage in the important stages of:

- naming the problem and exploring how others name the problem
- identifying conflicts of interest (interpreted broadly) that may influence responses to the problem
- locating the duties owed to patients in ethical theory
- learning from, and sharing, the experience.

The law, professional guidance and policy provide an unequivocal starting point: inaction in the face of justifiable concerns about a colleague's performance is not an option. However, to travel ethically and defensibly from this unequivocal starting point remains challenging: I hope this chapter contributes to making that journey easier.

References

1 Levi P. *Other People's Trades*. R Rosenthal, translator. London: Abacus Books; 1990.

2 There is a considerable literature on the meaning of competence and its relationship to performance. However in this chapter, I am using the word 'performance' (what a doctor does) as a broad process by which observers assess a doctor's competence (and perhaps other traits or behaviours unrelated to a narrow definition of competence).

3 The Stationery Office. *Report of the Inquiry into Quality and Practice Within the National Health Service Arising from the Actions of Rodney Ledward*. London: The Stationery Office; 2001; *Learning from Bristol: the report of the public inquiry into children's heart surgery at the Bristol Royal Infirmary 1984–95* (Command Paper: CM 520). http://www.bristol-inquiry.org.uk; 2001; *Fifth Report of the Shipman Inquiry – Safeguarding Patients: lessons from the past – proposals for the future* (Command Paper: CM 6394). http://www.shipman-inquiry.org.uk; 2004; *Report of the Kerr/Haslam Inquiry* (Command Paper: CM 6640). London: Department of Health; 2005.

4 Department of Health. *An Organisation with a Memory*. London: The Stationery Office; 2000; Department of Health. *Good Doctors, Safer Patients: Proposals to Strengthen the System to Assure and Improve the Performance of Doctors and to Protect the Safety of Patients: A Report by the Chief Medical Officer*. London: The Stationery Office; 2006.

5 Rosenthal M. *The Incompetent Doctor: behind closed doors*. Buckingham: Open University Press; 1996.

6 For a detailed review of the relevant legislation (including amendments) that determines the work of the GMC, *see* http://www.gmc-uk.org/index.htm (accessed 3 August 2005).

7 For two detailed examinations of the GMC's work, *see* Stacey M. *Regulating British Medicine: the General Medical Council*. Chichester: Wiley & Sons; 1992; Smith RG. *Medical Discipline: the professional conduct jurisdiction of the General Medical Council 1858–1990* (Oxford Socio-Legal Studies Series). Oxford: Clarendon Press; 1994.

8 GMC. http://www.gmc-uk.org/register/default.htm (accessed 3 August 2005).

9 GMC. *Duties of a Doctor*. http://www.gmc-uk.org/standards/default.htm (accessed 3 August 2005).

10 GMC. http://www.gmc-uk.org/med_ed/default.htm (accessed 4 August 2005).

11 GMC. http://www.gmc-uk.org/probdocs/default.htm (accessed 4 August 2005).

12 The CHRE was established by the National Health Service Reform and Health Care Professions Act 2002. It was originally known as the Council for the Regulation of Health Care Professionals. For further information on its work, *see* http://www.chre.org.uk

13 The meaning of 'undue leniency' was considered in *Ruscillo v Council for the Regulation of Healthcare Professionals and General Medical Council* [2004] EWCA Civ 1356; *Council for the Regulation of Healthcare Professionals v Nursing and*

Midwifery Council and Truscott (General Medical Council intervening) [2005] 1 WLR 717, CA.

14 Esmail A. GMC and the future of revalidation: failure to act on good intentions. *BMJ*. 2005; **330**: 1144–7; Baker R. After Shipman: why so little progress? 11 May 2006; http://saferhealthcare.org.uk/IHI/Topics/SafetyCulture/Literature/AfterShipman. htm (accessed 15 June 2006); Smith J. What are we doing post Shipman in the UK? Lecture at the Royal Society of Medicine One Day Conference *After Shipman: Trust Between Doctors and Patients*. Tuesday 2 May 2006.

15 The Report contains 44 recommendations in total.

16 For an analysis of the way in which clinical governance relates to ethics and standards of healthcare, *see* Campbell A. Clinical governance: watch word or buzz word? *J Med Ethics*. 2001; **27**: i54–6.

17 Institute of Health Services Management. *Clinical Governance: clinician, heal thyself?* (Policy Document). London: Institute of Health Services Management; 1998.

18 For a description of the ways in which whistle-blowers can be treated, *see* Hunt G. A dozen ways to shoot the messenger. In: Hunt G, ed. *Whistleblowing in the Health Service: accountability, law and professional practice*. London: Edward Arnold; 1995; pp. 155–8; Faunce T, Bolsin S, Chan WP. Supporting whistleblowers in academic medicine: training and respecting the courage of professional conscience. *J Med Ethics*. 2004; **30**: 40–3.

19 *Bolam v Friern Management Committee*. [1957] 2 *All ER* 118.

20 Stacey M. Medical accountability. In: Hunt G, ed. *Whistleblowing in the Health Service: accountability, law and professional practice*. London: Edward Arnold; 1995. pp. 36–7.

21 Samanta A, Samana J. Legal Standard of Care: a shift from the traditional Bolam test. *Clin Med*. 2003; **3**(5): 443–6.

22 *Bolitho v City & Hackney Heath Authority*. [1997] 3 *WLR* 583.

23 Teff H. The standard of care in medical negligence – moving on from Bolam? *Oxford J Legal Studies*. 1998; **18**(3): 473–84; Brazier M, Miola J. Bye-bye Bolam: a medical litigation revolution? [2000] 8 *Med LR* 85–114; Khan M. Bolitho – claimant's friend or enemy? *Med Law*. 2001; **20**(4): 483–91; McHale J. Quality in healthcare: a role for the law? *Qual Saf Health Care*. 2002; **11**(1): 88–91; Samanta A, Samana J. *Ibid*.

24 For comment on the types of situations in which an expert opinion may be rejected by a judge, *see Med Law Mon*. 1998; **4**(10): 4–5.

25 McHale J. Quality in healthcare: a role for the law? *Qual Saf Health Care*. 2002; **11**(1): 88.

26 McHale J. *Ibid*.

27 Vincent CA, Young M, Phillips A. Why do people sue their doctors? A study of patients and relatives taking action. *The Lancet*. 1994; **343**: 1609–13.

28 Brazier M. *Medicine, Patients and the Law*. 1st ed. London: Penguin; 1992. Ch. 16.

29 Rosenthal M. *Ibid*.

30 For example, the GMC, BMA and several Royal Colleges have all published guidance on end-of-life decision-making: *see*, for example, GMC. *Withholding and*

Withdrawing Life-prolonging Treatments: good practice in decision-making. London: GMC; 2002; BMA. *Withholding and Withdrawing Life-prolonging Treatment.* London: BMA; 2000; Royal College of Paediatrics and Child Health. *Withholding or Withdrawing Life Sustaining Treatment in Children: a framework for practice.* 2nd ed. London: RCPCH; 2004.

31 GMC. *Duties of a Doctor and Good Medical Practice.* 3rd ed. http://www.gmc-uk.org/standards/default.htm; 2001.

32 RCGP. *Good Medical Practice for General Practitioners.* London: RCGP; 2002.

33 RCGP. *Policy Statement: quality indicators in general practice.* http://www.rcgp.org.uk/corporate/position/qualityindicators.pdf; 2002 (accessed 5 August 2005).

34 RCGP. *Portfolio of Evidence of Professional Standards for the Revalidation of General Practitioners.* http://www.rcgp.org.uk/press/docs/revalidation/pdf; 2004 (accessed 5 August 2005).

35 RCGP. *Toolkit for Managing GPs who may have a Performance Problem.* London: RCGP (St Paul's Quality Unit); 2001.

36 Department of Health. *The NHS Plan: a plan for investment, a plan for reform.* London: Department of Health; Cm 4818–I; 2000.

37 Department of Health. *Reconfiguring the Department of Health's Arm's Length Bodies.* http://www.dh.gov.uk/assetRoot/04/09/81/36/04098136.pdf; 2004 (accessed 5 August 2005).

38 Pollock AM. *NHS Plc: the privatisation of our health care.* London: Verso; 2004.

39 Pellegrino ED, Thomasma DC. *The Virtues in Medical Practice.* New York: Oxford University Press; 1993.

40 Jacob J. *Doctors and Rules.* London: Routledge; 1988.

41 Chambers T. Framing our mistakes. In: Rubin SB, Zoloth L, eds. *Margin of Error: the ethics of mistakes in the practice of medicine.* Hagerstown, MD: University Publishing Group; 2000.

42 Brennan TA *et al.* Incidence of adverse events and negligence in hospitalized patients. *New Eng J Med.* 1991; **324**: 370–6; Leape LL. Error in medicine. *JAMA.* 1994; **272**(23): 1851–7; Berwick DM. A primer on leading the improvement of systems. *BMJ.* 1996; **312**: 619–22.

43 Hilfiker D. Facing our mistakes. *New Eng J Med.* 1984; **310**: 2; Christensen JF, Levinson W, Dunn PM. The heart of darkness: the impact of perceived mistakes on physicians. *J Gen Int Med.* 1992; **7**: 424–31; Fonsecka C. To err was fatal. *BMJ.* 1996; **313**: 1640–2; Frader JE. Mistakes in medicine: personal and moral responses. In: Rubin SB, Zoloth L, eds. *Margin of Error: the ethics of mistakes in the practice of medicine.* Hagerstown, MD: University Publishing Group; 2000.

44 Senders JW, Moray NP. *Human Error: cause, prediction and reduction.* Hillsdale, NJ: Lawrence Erlbaum; 1991; Makeham MAB *et al.* An international taxonomy for errors in general practice. *Med J Australia.* 2002; **177**(2): 68–72; Dovey SM *et al.* A preliminary taxonomy of medical errors in family practice. *Qual Saf Health Care.* 2002; **11**: 233–8.

45 Cassell E. *The Nature of Suffering and the Goals of Medicine.* New York: Oxford University Press; 1991.

46 Pringle M, Wilson T, Grol R. Measuring 'goodness' in individuals and health-care systems. *BMJ*. 2002; **325**: 704–7; Campbell SM *et al*. Improving the quality of healthcare: research methods used in developing and applying quality indicators in primary care. *BMJ*. 2003; **326**: 816–19.

47 Firth-Cozens J, Payne R, eds. *Stress in Health Professionals: psychological and organisational causes and interventions*. Chichester: John Wiley & Sons; 1999; Mandell H, Spiro H, eds. *When Doctors Get Sick*. Dordrecht: Kluwer Academic; 2003.

48 Freidson E. *The Profession of Medicine*. Chicago: University of Chicago Press; 1970; Sharpe VA, Faden AI. *Medical Harm: historical, conceptual and ethical dimensions of iatrogenic illness*. Cambridge: Cambridge University Press; 1998; Rosenthal M, Mulcahy L, Lloyd-Bostock S, eds. *Medical Mishaps: pieces of the puzzle*. Buckingham: Open University Press; 1999; Freidson E. *Professionalism: the third logic*. Cambridge: Polity Press; 2001; Mulcahy L. *Disputing Doctors: the socio-legal dynamics of complaints about medical care*. Buckingham: Open University Press; 2004.

49 Bosk C. *Forgive and Remember: managing medical failure*. Chicago: University of Chicago Press; 1979; Wu AW *et al*. Do house officers learn from their mistakes? *JAMA*. 1991; **265**: 2089–94.

50 Helman C. Disease and pseudo-disease: a case history of pseudo-angina. In: Hahn RA, Gaines AD, eds. *Physician of Western Medicine: anthropological approaches to theory and practice*. Dordrecht: Reidel; 1985.

51 Rosenthal M. *Ibid*.

52 Greenhalgh T, Hurwitz B. Why study narrative? *BMJ*. 1999; **318**: 48–50; Greenhalgh T. Narrative-based medicine in an evidence-based world. *BMJ*. 1999; **318**: 323–5; Greenhalgh T. *Narrative-based Primary Care: a practical guide*. Oxford: Radcliffe Medical Press; 2002.

53 Kuhn T. *The Structure of Scientific Revolutions*. Chicago: University of Chicago Press; 1962.

54 Mol A. *The Body Multiple: ontology in medical practice*. Durham, NC: Duke University Press; 2002.

55 Atkinson P. *Medical Work and Medical Talk*. London: Sage; 1995.

56 Hughes E. *Men and Their Work*. New York: The Free Press; 1958.

57 Foucault M. *The Birth of the Clinic*. London: Routledge; 1976.

58 Cited in: Sinclair S. *Making Doctors: an institutional apprenticeship*. Oxford: Berg; 1997. p. 24.

59 McKay AC. Supererogation and the profession of medicine. *J Med Ethics*. 2002; **28**: 70–3; Downie R. Supererogation and altruism: a comment. *J Med Ethics*. 2002; **28**: 75–6.

60 Fox R. Training for uncertainty. In: Merton R, Reader G, Kendall P, eds. *The Student Physician*. Cambridge, MA: Harvard University Press; 1957.

61 Dowrick C. Uncertainty and responsibility. In: Dowrick C, Frith L, eds. *General Practice and Ethics: uncertainty and responsibility*. London: Routledge; 1999; Willis J. *Friends in Low Places*. Oxford: Radcliffe Medical Press; 2001; Green C, Holden J. Diagnostic uncertainty in general practice: a unique opportunity for research? *Eur J Gen Prac*. 2003; **9**(1): 13–15; RCGP. *The Future of General*

Practice: a statement by the Royal College of General Practitioners. London: RCGP; 2004; Dew K *et al.* The glorious twilight of uncertainty. *Soc Sci & Med.* 2005; **61**(6): 1189–200.

62 Haslam D. 'Schools and hospitals' for 'education and health'. *BMJ.* 2003; **326**: 234–5.

63 Ashcroft RE. Bioethics and conflicts of interest. *Stud Hist & Phil Biol & Biomed Sci.* 2004; **13**: 20–27.

64 Rodwin MA. *Medicine, Money and Morals: physicians' conflicts of interest.* New York: Oxford University Press; 1995.

65 Martin JP. *Hospitals in Trouble.* Oxford: Blackwell; 1985; Pilgrim D. Explaining abuse and inadequate care. In: Hunt G, ed. *The Health Service: accountability, law and professional practice.* London: Edward Arnold; 1995.

66 Firth-Cozens J. The psychological problems of doctors. In: Firth-Cozens J, Payne R, eds. *Stress in Health Professionals: psychological and organisational causes and interventions.* Chichester: John Wiley & Sons; 1999.

67 Firth-Cozens J. *Ibid.* p. 85.

68 Rosenthal M. *Ibid.*

69 General Medical Council. *Doctors Should Not Treat Themselves or their Families.* London: GMC; 1998; BMA. *Ethical Responsibilities in Treating Doctors who are Patients: guidance from the ethics department.* London: BMA; 2004.

70 Department of Health. *Supporting Doctors, Protecting Patients: a consultation paper on preventing, recognising and dealing with poor clinical performance of doctors in the NHS in England.* London: Department of Health; 1999. para. 2.44.

71 Chambers R, Belcher J. Self-reported healthcare over the past ten years: a survey of general practitioners. *BJGP.* 1992; **42**: 153–6; Nuffield Provincial Hospitals Trust. *The Provision of Medical Services to Sick Doctors: a conspiracy of friendliness?* London: NPHT; 1994; Thompson WT *et al.* Challenge of culture, conscience and contract to general practitioners' care of their own health: qualitative study. *BMJ.* 2001; **323**: 728–31.

72 National Clinical Assessment Authority. *Understanding Performance Difficulties in Doctors: an NCAA report.* London: NCAA; 2004.

73 Sources include the BMA Counselling Service http://www.bma.org.uk, the National Counselling Service for Sick Doctors http://www.ncssd.org.uk, the Sick Doctors Trust http://www.sick-doctors-trust.co.uk and the Doctors' Support Network http://www.dsn.org.uk

74 Livingstone K. Three ways to make us all safer. *The Guardian*, 4 August 2005.

75 Kultgen J. *Ethics and Professionalism.* Philadelphia: University of Pennsylvania Press; 1988; pp. 136–52; Stacey M. Medical accountability. In: Hunt G, ed. *The Health Service: accountability, law and professional practice.* London: Edward Arnold; 1995.

76 Godlee F. The GMC: out of its depth? *BMJ.* 2005; **331**; Horton R. A dismal and dangerous verdict against Roy Meadow. *The Lancet.* 2005; **366**: 277–8.

77 Although Dworkin uses the term 'trumping' in relation to rights; *see* Dworkin R. *Taking Rights Seriously.* London: Gerald Duckworth; 1977.

78 General Medical Council. *Duties of a Doctor. Ibid.*

79 General Medical Council. *Good Medical Practice. Ibid.*

80 http://www.ncas.npsa.nhs.uk

81 Hunt G. Introduction: whistleblowing and the breakdown of accountability. In: Hunt G, ed. *The Health Service: accountability, law and professional practice.* London: Edward Arnold; 1995. p. xiii.

82 Rosenthal M. *Ibid.* pp. 14–19.

83 Pinkus RL. Learning to keep a cautious tongue: the reporting of mistakes in neurosurgery 1890–1930. In: Rubin SB, Zoloth L, eds. *Margin of Error: the ethics of mistakes in the practice of medicine.* Hagerstown, MD: University Publishing Group; 2000.

84 Bosk C. *Forgive and Remember: managing medical failure.* Chicago: University of Chicago Press; 1979.

Chapter 11

Ethics support and education in primary care

Anne Slowther and Michael Parker

Far best is he who knows all things himself;
Good, he that hearkens when men counsel right;
But he who neither knows, nor lays to heart
Another's wisdom, is a useless wight.

Aristotle (quoting Hesiod)[1]

Introduction

The increasing awareness of, and interest in, ethical issues in healthcare in recent years has raised the question of what knowledge, skills and experience health professionals have to enable them to engage with these often difficult decisions or situations. What ethics education is provided for health professionals in training and what are the sources of support, advice and education when they are facing ethical difficulties in their practice? Perhaps more importantly, what ethics education and support should be available to health professionals? In this chapter, we will consider these questions with particular reference to the context of primary care, drawing on the experience of ethics education and support in secondary care where appropriate.

Ethics in healthcare practice

Health professionals encounter ethical issues in their work on a daily basis. Sometimes these are explicitly acknowledged. Should we withdraw ventilation or nutrition from this patient? Should I pass on information about this person's HIV status to his or her spouse? More often, however, they are recognised rather more implicitly as part of the complexity of day-to-day clinical practice and only infrequently addressed more explicitly. Do I share this information with the wider healthcare team? Does this patient really understand the risks and benefits of treatment sufficiently well to make an informed choice? How do I balance the competing needs of different patients?

When health professionals are troubled by these ethical concerns, perhaps as a result of differences of opinion within the healthcare team or perhaps because of a perceived conflict between important moral values, they can often feel the need for advice or guidance. In many cases, health professionals will turn first to more experienced colleagues for advice. In others they will seek advice and guidance from a range of external sources, including professional guidelines such as those produced by the GMC, professional organisations such as the BMA or perhaps from defence unions.

The initial concern of health professionals when confronted by a difficult decision raising ethical issues will often, understandably, be to seek clarity, perhaps from one of the above sources, about the relevant law and professional guidelines. These can provide an essential framework for understanding what constitutes good practice, by articulating the underlying principles that guide practice and by setting limits on what is permissible. What such laws and guidelines do not provide, however, in most cases is a determinative answer to the question of what the health professional should do in any particular situation.

There is good reason for this. Behaving ethically in a particular case when dealing with a particular patient requires more than knowledge of abstract principles, general guidelines or statute and case law. It involves, in addition, the application and interpretation of these in the light of understanding and experience of a specific context such as an individual case or healthcare setting. That is, it requires clinically informed moral judgment. Thus GMC guidelines on confidentiality, for example, say that a doctor is allowed to breach confidentiality where he or she is concerned about harms to a third party if there is a 'risk of death or serious harm',[2] but the interpretation of what counts as a 'risk of death' or a 'serious harm' in a particular case requires a judgment by the doctor making the decision, a judgment he or she must be prepared to justify in relation to the specifics of the case, in court if necessary.

This suggests that in practical decision-making in difficult ethical situations healthcare professionals will, in addition to general guidance, need education and support to help them think through the particularities of the case in the light of such guidance. The increasing number of enquiries to the BMA ethics unit and the findings of surveys of health professionals reflect this and suggest that it is this specific support, often provided in a multidisciplinary setting by their peers, that health professionals value most when confronted with ethical issues.[3, 4] In some settings recognition of the needs of health professionals has led to the establishment, often by those health professionals themselves, of innovative forms of ethics support and advice in the local healthcare setting.[5] These developments are discussed below.

A key complementary question raised by the considerations above concerns how health professionals can best be equipped with the ethical awareness, skills and support they need to enable them to identify and deal with the implicit and explicit ethical issues in their day-to-day practice and to interpret professional and legal guidelines in the context of specific situations. The General Medical Council (GMC) has, since 1993, recognised that high quality, clinically-based ethics education in both undergraduate training and continuing professional development is key in this regard.[6] Interestingly, however, a recent survey of specialist registrars conducted for the Royal College of Physicians (RCP) found that one third of respondents reported that they had never had clinical ethics education or training.[7] What this suggests, in combination with the above, is that while ethics education in the medical curriculum is essential, this is likely to need to be complemented by both ongoing professional education and appropriate, locally-based ethics support.

The question of what types of ethics support and education are most appropriate in different healthcare settings is an important one. It is unlikely to be the case that the same model will be useful or feasible everywhere. A key distinction in this respect, in UK healthcare, is that between primary and secondary care. The growth of awareness of ethical issues in healthcare has, until recently, largely been driven by concern about ethical issues arising in acute medicine in the hospital setting, for example, end-of-life decision-making, ethics in intensive care and so on. But ethical issues also arise in primary care and the hospital clinical ethics committee, or some variant of it, is unlikely to be an appropriate mechanism for ethics support in many primary care settings. In this chapter, we look at the history of the development of ethics support and education and consider the relationship between the ethical issues arising in secondary and primary care. We argue, using examples, that primary care presents ethical issues that are different in important respects and that the context in which primary healthcare is provided is significantly and relevantly different to secondary care. In the light of this, we go on to look at what forms of ethics support and education would be most appropriate for the primary care setting. We begin, however, by briefly describing the development of clinical ethics support and education.

The development of ethics education and clinical ethics support

Ethics education

Ethics has, for as long as medicine has been practised, constituted an important aspect of medical training and practice. In some cases, the ethical component of such training was made explicit, for example, by reference to the Hippocratic oath or through discussion of the demand to 'first do no harm'. Even where ethics education was not explicit, however, the hidden curriculum of the medical education received by trainee doctors, either on the firm or in their first years of practice has always been, and continues to be, permeated by an important and all-pervading ethical or moral dimension. Despite the longstanding recognition of the importance of ethics in medicine, until quite recently, explicit and organised teaching of ethics by qualified teachers was very patchy, with some students receiving very little.

A significant change in this respect began to occur in the 1960s and 70s. A major early influence came from the London Medical Group, a conglomeration of medical student societies, organised under the guidance of Edward Shotter of the Student Christian Movement. By the mid-1970s, most medical schools had such a group. These groups were behind several initiatives to create an explicit presence for ethics and communication skills teaching on the medical curriculum. From the London and Edinburgh Medical Groups came the Institute of Medical Ethics which, with GMC encouragement, investigated the teaching of medical ethics in UK medical schools and published its findings in the 1987 Pond Report. This was followed, some five years later, by the publication by the GMC of *Tomorrow's Doctors* in 1993,[6] which required education in ethics to be a core component of medical education in all UK medical schools.

In 1998, a consortium of medical ethics teachers in UK medical schools published a consensus statement setting out a core curriculum.[8] Currently all medical courses include a substantial ethics component.[7] The content and extent of this teaching varies significantly from school to school and in no case is the very extensive and probably unachievable 'core curriculum' set out in the 1998 document covered in its entirety. Nevertheless, the ethics curriculum can in some cases be quite extensive. Topics taught in the Oxford medical school curriculum, for example, include: confidentiality, consent, ethical issues at the end of life, genetic testing, medical research, treating children, reproductive ethics, psychiatry and treating patients without their consent, some ward-based ethics teaching around real cases and a one-month special study module for students with a particular interest.

Clinical ethics support

The development of formal models of ethics support for health professionals in clinical practice has, until recently, been more widespread in North America than in other healthcare systems. Clinical ethics committees and clinical ethicists are well established in American hospitals, largely because the accreditation requirements of large health insurers mean that healthcare institutions must have a mechanism for addressing the ethical issues arising in patient care.[9] In the US, there is a very clear distinction between clinical ethics committees and research ethics committees (IRBs). In many European countries by contrast, but not in the UK, clinical ethics support has developed within a model of combined research/clinical ethics committees. Some European countries have legal requirements for hospitals to have a committee that addresses the ethical issues arising in both clinical practice and research within the institution.[10] More recently, there has been a trend to separate clinical ethics committees from research ethics committees as recognition of the ethical difficulties facing health professionals in clinical practice has increased.[11] In recent years, there has been an increase in the number of clinical ethicists in some European countries, although the number is still very small compared to North America.

In the UK, where clinical and research ethics committees have always had completely different functions, there has been a rapid expansion of clinical ethics committees in secondary and tertiary care settings from 20 in 2000 to 75 in 2005.[12] The development of these committees, often initiated by health professionals themselves, has largely been *ad hoc* and bottom-up. Many of these committees have an ethicist as a member of the committee, but very few hospitals have an ethicist whose role extends outside the committee structure.[13]

The focus of clinical ethics support in all countries where it has developed has been very much hospital-based and concerned with issues arising in acute medicine. There are *some* examples of clinical ethics committees in community hospitals in the US and in nursing homes in the Netherlands, but these are still institutionally based committees. There is very little evidence of clinical ethics support in primary care, although one or two primary care trusts (PCTs) in the UK have now established a clinical ethics committee[14] and some hospital-based committees consider cases referred by local GPs.

What are clinical ethics committees?

Clinical ethics committees are essentially advisory bodies that provide support and guidance to clinicians, healthcare managers and patients and their families in dealing with the difficult ethical issues that can arise in providing good patient care. Their role is to support those making difficult decisions rather than taking responsibility for the making of such decisions. A key characteristic of most committees is that they are multidisciplinary and have lay membership, thus bringing a range of perspectives and values to the issues they consider.[15] An individual ethicist does not provide this broad range of perspectives but has specific knowledge and skills in ethical decision-making, can be more flexible than a committee in responding to urgent cases and may also be in a better position to develop long-term supportive relationships with the clinical setting. An ethicist and an ethics committee are complementary and not an either/or option for an organisation.[16, 17]

What do clinical ethics committees and clinical ethicists do?

Most descriptions of the role of clinical ethics committees specify three main functions of the committee.

1. Providing advice and support in individual cases.

2. Providing advice on the ethical implications of policies and guidelines relating to patient care developed by the institution.

3. Facilitating education of health professionals within the institution on ethical issues relating to patient care.

This is a broad, and somewhat daunting, remit for a single committee or ethicist and in practice most committees focus predominantly on one or two of the functions, usually individual case consultation or input into institutional policy.

Does ethics support make a difference to patient care?

There is surprisingly little evidence on the effectiveness of clinical ethics committees and clinical ethicists, which may be partly explained by the difficulty in defining outcome measures in ethics. It may be possible to demonstrate whether health professionals find such support useful in their practice or if ethics committees make a difference to clinician behaviour, but whether that change results in improved (i.e. more ethical) patient care is a more difficult question to answer. From the limited evidence available we can say that health professionals perceive a need for clinical ethics support,[7, 18] that those clinicians who refer cases to a clinical ethics committee or ethicist express satisfaction with the process[19–22] and that ethics case consultation has been shown to change clinical practice in the specific context of withholding and withdrawing treatment in the intensive care setting.[23–25] There is a need for further evaluation of current models of clinical ethics support and for exploration of alternative models that may be more appropriate for different healthcare settings such as primary care.

What is special about ethics in primary care?

We have argued that the growth of ethics education in the medical school curriculum and of clinical ethics committees has, for the most part, been driven by concerns about the kinds of issues arising in the acute hospital setting: consent to surgery, end-of-life decision-making, critical care, organ transplantation and so on. This has led to a growth in ethics support largely within and predominantly oriented towards the acute hospital setting. More recently, however, there has been a growing interest in the ethical issues arising in primary care and recognition of the need for education and ethics support for family doctors and other primary care professionals. What would an appropriate form of ethics support and education for primary care look like? In addressing this question, we will first consider what, if any, are the special, unique ethical issues or emphases in primary care. Using case examples, we investigate the distinctive ethical issues arising within primary care practice itself. We also explore the ethical implications of the organisational location of primary care provision. In the light of these reflections, we go on to discuss some key features of an ethics support and education appropriate for primary care.

The social context of primary care and its implications for clinical ethics education and support

There are clear practical reasons why clinical ethics support in primary care might require a different model from that in secondary or tertiary care. In the UK the traditional structure of primary care, and more specifically general practice, means that individual doctors and nurses work independently, making decisions about patient care often without the monitoring and support structures provided within the hospital setting. This may result in a lack of awareness of ethical issues arising in practice, fewer opportunities for discussion with colleagues and difficulty in developing workable processes for providing ethics support. The establishment of PCTs in the UK has provided a more formal organisational structure for primary care, but individual clinical units, such as GP practices or community health centres, are still geographically dispersed and this will continue to create barriers for easy referral to a central committee or a rapid response from an ethicist.

A more fundamental question for those wishing to develop clinical ethics support in primary care, and one that also applies to development of ethics education in primary care, relates to the content of the support/education rather than the delivery process. Are the ethical issues that arise in primary care, and the approaches used to resolve these issues, different from those in secondary and tertiary care; and if they are, what are the implications for ethics education and support? Several authors have argued that the different conceptual frameworks of primary and secondary care, and the different settings in which healthcare is delivered, will influence both the type of ethical dilemma experienced and the approach to dealing with it.[26-29] The concept of primary care is one of accessible, first contact and continuing care with an emphasis on long-term relationships, community and preventive healthcare, and the health professional as advocate of the patient in the wider healthcare system. The concept of secondary and tertiary care is one of technology-based individualistic, short-term care, with an emphasis on cure of specific diseases and the health professional as specialist in a specific disease or system. It is likely that the more individualistic model of secondary and tertiary care will place a greater emphasis on autonomy and individual rights than the more social model of primary care. Also, the structure and setting of primary care may mean that the range of ethical issues, or the frequency with which specific issues are encountered, differs from secondary and tertiary care. Working with families and at the health/social care interface, dealing with diagnostic uncertainty, and maintaining interdisciplinary professional relationships are more likely to be the source of ethical problems than discontinuing life-prolonging treatment or balancing the risk of harm and benefit in novel treatments. Empirical ethics studies in primary care, although fairly small in number, provide support for this hypothesis, identifying issues such as relationships with colleagues,[30] conflicts of interest[31] and resource allocation.[32] Studies focusing on single issues suggest that they are interpreted differently in different contexts, for example, patients' views on confidentiality of medical records differ depending on whether the context is primary or secondary care.[33] A strong message from these studies, and from studies that look at the process of moral decision-making in primary care, is the importance of context and relationships in the identification of ethical issues and methods of resolving them.[34-36] This contrasts with a more abstract principlist approach, which characterises much of traditional medical ethics discussion and teaching.

This is not to say that ethical principles are not important in primary care. Professional codes of conduct and guidelines on issues such as consent and confidentiality carry obligations for all health professionals whatever their sphere of work and principles such as respect for autonomy, acting in the patient's best interests and behaving fairly are fundamental to good clinical practice at all levels. However, the translation of these principles into the day-to-day encounters between patients and health professionals will be shaped by the context in which the encounters take place. Doyal has argued that the traditional view of medical ethics is closely linked to the practice of acute medicine in the hospital setting.[28] Thus, respect for autonomy is manifest in the practice of informed consent to treatment with a focus on assessment of competence, provision of information and individual treatment decisions. In primary care, formalised informed consent processes are less common. Specific situations, such as performing minor surgical procedures or immunisation of children, may involve a process comparable to consent for surgery in secondary care, including a signed consent recorded in the notes (although in the case of minor surgery, written consent is not universally obtained in primary care). However, many healthcare decisions in primary care are not discrete isolated choices about individual treatments. They are often about long-term commitment to chronic disease management and preventive measures, including lifestyle changes, set against a background of changing medical knowledge and patient experience. A decision to refuse treatment or follow medical advice in these situations does not result in a termination of the clinical relationship as it often does in secondary care (if I decline to have the surgical treatment recommended for my condition, having considered all the information, then there is little point in my continuing attendance at the surgical clinic). The nature of primary care is one of an ongoing relationship between clinician and patient whatever the outcome of an individual treatment decision (if I decline treatment of my hypertension recommended by my GP, I will still continue to see the same GP for other problems or even to request that he or she monitor my blood pressure from time to time). Respect for autonomy in this context involves something broader than a formal consent process. It involves providing opportunities to revisit the decision at other times when the patient consults to allow for changing patient views and experiences over time. A man with diabetes whose wife is dying of breast cancer and who has two small children to care for may decline to follow the advice to maintain tight glycaemic control by frequent blood sugar monitoring and adjustment of his insulin. A year after his wife's death, with both children settled at school, he may respond more positively to suggestions that he puts more focus on his diabetes management. It may involve helping patients with other problems that are restricting their ability to make an autonomous decision about their treatment. A woman whose life is completely dominated by the difficulties of caring for a parent with Alzheimer's disease and a son who has attention deficit disorder may not wish to attend hypertension clinics and give up smoking. If respite care for her parent and appropriate support for her son can be provided, she may be able to focus more on her own health and make different decisions.

This broader concept of respect for autonomy is possible in primary care because of two key features of primary care – continuity of care and direct access to care. In this context GPs, community nurses, health visitors and other primary care professionals often have knowledge of their patients' situations beyond the immediate clinical problems and are often also caring for other members of the patients' families. They also have multiple contacts with patients for a wider range of reasons, not restricted to a single clinical condition. This provides an opportunity but also creates a responsibility to move beyond the narrow informed consent model of treatment. A further feature of primary care is that of family care. In many cases a primary care clinician, for example a GP or health visitor, will care for several members of a family. Community nurses will often care for a patient in their own home, sharing care with family members. Decisions made by an individual patient may have huge implications for other members of their family, to whom the GP or nurse may also have a duty of care. Thus a focus on the individual patient and their autonomous wishes may not always be as straightforward as it is perceived in secondary care, where usually the clinicians do not have to deal with the implications of patients' decisions on others.

Empirical work on ethical decision-making in primary care, including work by one of us,[37] suggests that the nature of the clinician–patient relationship in primary care is not that of a relationship governed by rigid, external moral rules; it is rather one in which ethical concerns arise out of specific relationships and situations. Shaped by the key features of primary care (continuity of care, open access care and family care), the nature of the ethical difficulties encountered and the ethical concepts used to resolve them are more complex and wide-ranging than those usually seen in the more circumscribed clinician–patient relationships that often occur in secondary care. We must be careful not to overplay the uniqueness of primary care in this respect, however. There are areas of secondary care, for example paediatrics, genetic and palliative care, where clinician–patient relationships are also set in a broader social context and strict adherence to a set of abstract moral rules does not capture the moral complexity of the situation. However, this broader social context to the clinician–patient relationship is core to primary care, particularly as it is structured in the UK, but is less universal in the secondary care setting. Below, we discuss two examples of cases in which the social dimension of the ethical aspects of primary care are obvious.

Ethics in primary care practice

> James Clarke is a 70-year-old man with dementia and chronic obstructive pulmonary disease. He is cared for at home by his 72-year-old wife. He has frequent chest infections for which he receives antibiotics and he requires oxygen at home. His most recent chest infection has not responded well to oral antibiotics and his general condition is deteriorating. He is not eating and is drinking little. He is unlikely to respond to more intensive treatment in hospital, but it is possible that with intravenous antibiotics and physiotherapy he may recover. Even if he recovers, he is likely to develop a similar infection again in the near future. Admission to hospital in the past has caused him distress because he does not cope well with changing environments. His wife says she thinks he should be in hospital.

Cases like this one will be familiar to many primary care clinicians. It illustrates the difficulties of making ethical decisions in situations of diagnostic uncertainty and social complexity. Important initial questions include how bad Mr Clarke's dementia is and whether he is able to express a preference about his treatment, how accurate the assumption that treatment is unlikely to be successful is, and what the likely effects on Mr Clarke and his wife are of him being admitted or staying at home. A standard ethical approach to this case would be to respect Mr Clarke's autonomous wishes regarding treatment if he was competent to make such a decision or, in the event that he was unable to make such a decision, to choose the course of action that would be in his best interests. Let us assume that Mr Clarke is unable to express his wishes regarding admission to hospital. His GP, Dr Jones, considers that it is not in his medical best interests to be admitted as he will become distressed and may well die in hospital. He may also die at home, but he will be in a familiar place with familiar people caring for him. But if Mr Clarke is to stay at home, his wife must make a commitment to care for him at a time when he may deteriorate and possibly die, a commitment that she may be unable or unwilling to make. Where do her wishes and interests fit into the decision-making process? Even if she is not also a patient of Dr Jones, they will probably have developed a relationship based on their shared concern and care for her husband. Dr Jones may have a sense of responsibility for her welfare as well as that of her husband, which may create conflict with the specific duty of care to act in Mr Clarke's best interests. Even if Mrs Clarke's specific interests are ignored and the focus remains on her husband, the question arises as to what role she has in determining his interests. In some healthcare systems, for example in the US, she would make the decision as his proxy on the assumption that she would best know his wishes and therefore make the decision he would make if he were able, thus respecting his autonomy. In the UK, proxy decision-making for incompetent adults is not the norm, although this may change with the introduction of the Mental Capacity Act 2005, which will allow a person to appoint someone to make decisions about their medical care if they become incompetent to make those decisions for themselves (lasting power of attorney).[38] However, even without such a legal power, Mrs Clarke will still have a crucial role in providing information about her husband's previously held beliefs and preferences, which will be important in assessing his best interests. In fact, it may be impossible to disentangle Mrs Clarke's interests from those of her husband. If the burden of care is too great and she is unable to cope with the situation, either physically or emotionally, her husband's quality of life will deteriorate. A further perspective in this case would be to consider where this specific decision fits within the narrative of Mr and Mrs Clarke's life together as a couple. Describing the decision in terms of a conflict between individual interests may not capture the more complex moral reality of family life.

The above discussion of the case of Mr Clarke is not a comprehensive ethical analysis but serves to demonstrate how the context of primary care can add moral complexity to medical decision-making, and the limitations of standard medical ethics approaches in dealing with these issues.

On the basis of a routine scan, Sarah Jones's first pregnancy was thought to be affected by a serious and fatal bone abnormality. When she was informed about this, Sarah discussed it with her husband and with her GP, Dr Lacey and decided to have a termination. Post-mortem examination revealed that the fetus had in fact been suffering from Asphyxiating Thoracic Dystrophy (ATD), a condition less severe than the bone disorder initially diagnosed but still fatal in 50% of cases. ATD is inherited as an autosomal recessive condition, meaning that the chance of a future fetus dying of the condition, if conceived by the same parents, is 12.5% because one in four of the parents' children would be affected and, of these, half would die. Sarah and her husband were given this advice at an appointment

Continued

with the genetic counsellor and were told that there is currently no genetic test for this condition. This information was also passed on to Dr Lacey.

Three weeks later Dr Lacey received a letter from Sarah, in which she informed her that her husband was very unlikely to have been the biological father of the fetus. In the letter she made it clear that although she thought this information might be important for the GP, she did not want it to be shared with her husband. She thought it likely that they would separate soon.

Cases like this one highlight both the social and familial nature of practice in primary care and the ethical significance of the relationships between health professionals in primary care and those in other services, in this case clinical genetics. The requirement to work closely with and to make negotiated decisions, often with an ethical dimension, with a range of healthcare or related services is a core feature of primary care practice. In any particular case, these other services might include social services, community mental health services, community nurses and health visitors as well as acute hospitals and hospital doctors. This multiprofessional context of ethical decision-making, while present in many other forms of healthcare, is at the heart of good practice in primary care.

In addition to raising questions about the appropriate relationship between different healthcare services, the case described above also presents a number of difficult ethical issues for the GP, arising out of the fact that she works with families. First, both Sarah and her husband are her patients and she will want, wherever possible, to ensure that they both have access to important healthcare information. At the same time, however, she will need to be concerned to make sure that she maintains the relationship of trust with her patients that will enable her to continue to support them in the future. The maintenance of long-term trusting relationships is clearly very important in primary care and this may be particularly important when there is the possibility that the patient, in this case Sarah, is very likely to need support, for example, around future pregnancies. This will mean that it will be important in the first instance to talk to Sarah about her reasons for not wanting this information disclosed and to ensure that Sarah understands the potential importance of this information for her husband. It will also be important to see whether it is possible to find a pragmatic and sensitive way of ensuring that this information is shared while also maintaining the trust of all concerned. It is not always possible in practice, however, to find a resolution that satisfies all parties and in such cases health professionals will need to consider the merits, both clinical and ethical, of the available alternatives and, in the light of these considerations and with reference to professional guidelines, make a moral judgment about which course of action to pursue. One way in which the need for moral judgment might arise in the case above would be if Sarah were to remain adamant that she did not want this information to be shared with her husband. Under such conditions, Dr Lacey would need to take into account a number of factors such as: When if ever is it acceptable to breach patient confidentiality in the interests of others, in this case Sarah's husband? What are the limits of the primary care doctor's responsibilities in such cases – to Sarah, to her husband? If she decides not to breach confidentiality, she will need to think carefully about what she ought to say to Sarah's husband next time he comes in, particularly if he asks specifically for reproductive advice in the light of the previously disclosed (inaccurate) information. What ought Dr Lacey to do if Sarah's husband's new partner presents to her for antenatal care? How much of this information should be passed on to the clinical genetics team? Each of these questions in its own way raises questions about the nature of the doctor–patient relationship in primary care and will require the doctor to do a number of things. She will need to:

- identify the options available and identify the moral and other arguments in favour and against each of these options
- consider the relative strength of these arguments, perhaps by talking to colleagues or, where it exists, to a clinical ethics committee
- make a judgment about which option to take in the light of counterarguments
- reflect on the outcome of whatever decision she ends up making (particularly if the decision was made on the basis of a consideration of the relative harms and benefits of the available options, and take this into account in future decision-making of this kind.

Like the case of Mr Clarke, the above discussion is not meant to constitute a comprehensive ethical analysis but simply to serve to indicate how the familial and long-term context of primary care can add moral complexity to medical decision-making, and the limitations of standard medical ethics approaches in dealing with these issues.

Organisational ethics in primary care

There has been an increasing interest in organisational healthcare ethics in North America in recent years and some UK clinical ethics committees in acute trusts are asked to advise on organisational issues such as the use of sponsorship and allocation of limited resources. With the creation of PCTs in the UK in 2000, a specific organisational structure was established to coordinate the delivery and commissioning of care for a local population. To the ethical difficulties faced by clinicians in primary care, we can now add the ethical difficulties faced by managers within PCTs (or other primary care organisations). Within the PCT structure, many of the managers are also local clinicians, who are often faced with ethical difficulties arising out of their dual roles. Any comprehensive development of education and support for ethical decision-making in primary care will need to involve a consideration of organisational ethics in this context.

A key ethical issue for all healthcare organisations, including those in primary care, is the question of a just distribution of limited healthcare resources. While resource allocation can also create ethical difficulties in individual clinician–patient relationships, it has not been the subject of ethical analysis and debate in this context to the same extent as issues such as consent and confidentiality. Issues of distributive justice are more commonly discussed by economists and those studying political philosophy, who are concerned with policy at a population level. The work of Norman Daniels,[39] and more recently Peter Singer and colleagues[40] has focused specifically on the ethics of resource allocation within healthcare organisations. Daniels' accountability for reasonableness framework emphasises the ethical significance of the process of decision-making and the communal basis of the decisions. This recognises that the organisational context of ethical decision-making calls for a different approach from standard medical ethics frameworks. Key factors for ethics education and support at an organisational level in primary care to consider will be the process of organisational decision-making, shared responsibility and theories of justice.

How can we develop ethics education and support in primary care?

We have identified a number of ways in which primary care differs from secondary care and have suggested, using cases, that as a result the kinds of ethical issues arising in primary care are likely to be different. This raises the issue of what would constitute an appropriate form of ethics support and education for primary care. In many cases, the ethical issues and concepts experienced by practitioners in primary care will be broadly similar to those described in the medical ethics literature that relates mainly to secondary care. Nevertheless, the specific issues that arise and the interpretation of key ethical concepts and principles are inevitably going to be shaped by the context of primary care, in particular the nature of relationships within primary care both with patients and with other services. We have suggested that, with rare exceptions, practitioners experience the ethical dimensions of their practice implicitly rather than explicitly and that resolution of ethical difficulties is a more complex process involving negotiation, reflection and review against a background of shared good practice, rather than application of external principles. A successful model of ethics support will need to work with these features of ethics experience in primary care.

At a clinical level, a model of support that works with practitioners rather than for practitioners is likely to be most effective by enabling practitioners to explicitly recognise and articulate the ethical issues that they implicitly deal with and by providing input into their process of decision-making. Possible ways in which this could be done include:

- introducing ethics input into current forums for sharing problems, such as clinical supervision and practice meetings
- working through case examples in standard educational sessions
- incorporating an ethical dimension into clinical guidelines that articulates the ethical dimension of the clinical decision
- setting up a forum/committee where more general issues can be discussed in order to inform the guidelines.

While the ultimate aim of ethics support at an organisational level in PCTs is likely to be, at least to some extent, to develop a shared ethical language and value set throughout the whole PCT organisation, a practical question for an ethics support service or programme must be where to start. It is clear from research carried out by one of us, that the issue of priority-setting and resource allocation raises the most immediate ethical concerns for PCTs. Many PCTs have specific committees or groups to decide on individual treatment requests outside the normally commissioned packages of care and, in some PCTs, these groups consider wider issues of priority-setting within the framework of the PCT's health improvement plan. This structural framework provides a natural starting place for developing a shared familiarity with, and use of, the underlying values that will inform these decisions. Having achieved this within these small groups, the exercise can then be rolled out throughout the organisation, including dialogue with patients' forums and partner organisations, such as the acute trusts.

Conclusions

In this chapter, we have explored some of the ethical issues arising in primary care. We have argued that many of these issues will be significantly different to those arising in acute, hospital-based medicine, partly because of the nature of primary healthcare practice and partly because of the institutional location of that practice. It is important not to overstate the differences between primary and secondary care, however. Many of the ethical issues arising will be very similar, or will at least have similar themes, to those in secondary care. Nevertheless, the differences are significant and we have argued that these differences will have important implications for the ways in which ethical issues are addressed and for the types of ethics support most appropriate for health professionals. At least three key differences seem particularly important. The first of these is the familial and social nature of primary care practice, which itself has two dimensions. It involves working with several members of the same family and it also involves working with patients and families, at least in some cases, for a significant period of their lives, i.e. over a number of years. The second of the key differences between primary and secondary care is the dispersed and often isolated, but community-based nature of practice. The third difference arises out of the direct role that PCTs have in questions of resource allocation.

These considerations, and the others we have discussed, suggest that primary care will require different forms of ethics support than those appropriate to other areas of medicine. It is probably premature to make specific recommendations on the provision of ethics education and support in primary care. A wider debate is needed that includes input from different clinical disciplines as well as ethicist and healthcare educators and evaluation of any new initiatives will be required. However, we can offer some suggestions to inform the debate.

- Undergraduate education in medical ethics should include consideration of the types of issue that are likely to arise in primary care and how the context of primary care shapes the experience of ethical decision-making by practitioners.
- Primary care practitioners (and managers) need access to ethics support and advice that is relevant to their day-to-day work; thus those providing support need to be familiar with the context of primary care.
- Ethics committees at an organisational level in primary care (for example in PCTs) may be more appropriate for advising on policies and guidelines rather than individual support. An individual ethicist model may work better for responding to individual difficulties and developing the ethical dimension of continuing professional development programmes.

The nature of primary care practice provides a useful reminder that ethical reflection needs to take into account the context in which healthcare practice is carried out and the important and central role of interpersonal relationships in healthcare. In addition to its importance in primary care, this is a useful reminder of the importance of context and relationships in the wider ethical dimension of healthcare.

References

1 Aristotle. *Nicomachean Ethics*. Ross, DW, translator. Book 1, Ch. 4. http://www.constitution.org/ari/ethic_01.htm#1.4

2 General Medical Council. *Confidentiality: protecting and providing information*. London: GMC; 2004.

3 Slowther A, Underwood M. Is there a demand for a clinical ethics advisory service in the UK? *J Med Ethics*. 1998; **24**(3): 207.

4 RCP Working Party on Clinical Ethics. *Ethics in Practice: background and recommendations for enhanced support*. London: RCP; 2005.

5 Slowther A, Bunch C, Woolnough B, Hope T. *Clinical Ethics Support Services in the UK: a review of the current position and likely development*. London: The Nuffield Trust; 2001.

6 General Medical Council. *Tomorrow's Doctors: recommendations on undergraduate medical education*. London: GMC; 2003.

7 RCP Working Party on Clinical Ethics. *Ibid*. pp. 31–4.

8 BMJ. Teaching medical ethics and law within medical education: a model for the UK core curriculum. *J Med Ethics*. 1998; **24**(3): 188–92.

9 Joint Commission for Accreditation of Healthcare Organisations. *Joint Commission for Healthcare Accreditation: comprehensive manual for hospitals*. Chicago: JAHO; 1996

10 Carbonell S, Scmitz P. Ethical function in Belgian hospital ethics committees: historical overview. In: Lebeer G, Moulin M, eds. *Ethical Function in Hospital Ethics Committees* (Biomed 2 Working Papers). Brussels: Universite Libre de Bruxelles; 2000. pp. 39–45.

11 van der Kloot Meijburg HH, ter Meulen RH. Developing standards for institutional ethics committees: lessons from The Netherlands. *J Med Ethics*. 2001; **27**(Suppl 1): i36-40.

12 UK Clinical Ethics Network. 2005. www.ethics-network.org.uk

13 Slowther A, Johnston C, Goodall J, Hope T. Development of clinical ethics committees. *BMJ*. 2004; **328**(7445): 950–2.

14 Clinical ethics committees in the UK. 2005. http://www.ethics-network.org.uk/Committee/list.htm

15 Slowther A, Bunch C, Woolnough B, Hope T. Clinical ethics support services in the UK: an investigation of the current provision of ethics support to health professionals in the UK. *J Med Ethics*. 2001; **27**(Suppl 1): i2–8.

16 Singer PA, Pellegrino ED, Siegler M. Ethics committees and consultants. *J Clin Ethics*. 1990; **1**(4): 263–7.

17 Slowther A, Johnston C, Goodall J, Hope T. *A Practical Guide for Clinical Ethics Support*. Oxford: The Ethox Centre; 2005. http://www.ethics-network.org.uk/reading/Guide/SectionA/sectionA.htm

18 Slowther A, Underwood M. Is there a demand for a clinical ethics advisory service in the UK? *J Med Ethics*. 1998; **24**(3): 207.

19 La PJ, Stocking CB, Silverstein MD, DiMartini A, Siegler M. An ethics consultation service in a teaching hospital. Utilization and evaluation. *JAMA*. 1988; **260**(6): 808–11.

20 La PJ, Stocking CB, Darling CM, Siegler M. Community hospital ethics consultation: evaluation and comparison with a university hospital service. *Am J Med*. 1992; **92**(4): 346–51.

21 Orr RD, Moon E. Effectiveness of an ethics consultation service. *J Fam Pract*. 1993; **36**(1): 49–53.

22 McClung JA, Kamer RS, DeLuca M, Barber HJ. Evaluation of a medical ethics consultation service: opinions of patients and healthcare providers. *Am J Med*. 1996; **100**(4): 456–60.

23 Schneiderman LJ, Gilmer T, Teetzel HD. Impact of ethics consultations in the intensive care setting: a randomized, controlled trial. *Critical Care Med*. 2000; **28**(12): 3920–4.

24 Schneiderman LJ, Gilmer T, Teetzel HD *et al*. Effect of ethics consultations on non-beneficial life-sustaining treatments in the intensive care setting: a randomized controlled trial. *JAMA*. 2003; **290**(9): 1166–72.

25 Dowdy MD, Robertson C, Bander JA. A study of proactive ethics consultation for critically and terminally ill patients with extended lengths of stay. *Critical Care Med*. 1998; **26**(2): 252–9.

26 Smith HL. Medical ethics in the primary care setting. *Soc Sci & Med*. 1987; **25**(6): 705–9.

27 Dickman RL. Family medicine and medical ethics – a natural and necessary union. *J Fam Practice*. 1980; **10**(4): 633–7.

28 Doyal L. Ethico-legal dilemmas within general practice. In: Dowrik C, Frith L, eds. *General Practice and Ethics: uncertainty and responsibility*. London: Routledge; 2005. pp. 45–61.

29 Fetters MD, Brody H. The epidemiology of bioethics. *J Clin Ethics*. 1999; **10**(2): 107–15.

30 Braunack-Mayer AJ. What makes a problem an ethical problem? An empirical perspective on the nature of ethical problems in general practice. *J Med Ethics*. 2001; **27**(2): 98–103.

31 Grumbach K, Osmond D, Vranizan K, Jaffe D, Bindman AB. Primary care physicians' experience of financial incentives in managed-care systems. *New Eng J Med*. 1998; **339**(21): 1516–21.

32 Ayres PJ. Rationing healthcare: views from general practice. *Soc Sci & Med*. 1996; **42**(7): 1021–5.

33 Carman D, Britten N. Confidentiality of medical records: the patient's perspective. *BJGP*. 1995; **45**(398): 485–8.

34 Rogers WA. Beneficence in general practice: an empirical investigation. *J Med Ethics*. 1999; **25**(5): 388–93.

35 Rogers WA. Whose autonomy? Which choice? A study of GPs' attitudes towards patient autonomy in the management of low back pain. *Fam Pract.* 2002; **19**(2): 140–5.

36 Christie RJ, Freer C, Hoffmaster CB, Stewart MA. Ethical decision making by British general practitioners. *J RCGP.* 1989; **39**(328): 448–51.

37 Slowther A. *Ethical Decision-making in Primary Care.* Oxford: Ethox Centre, University of Oxford; 2004.

38 Mental Capacity Act 2005. http://www.opsi.gov.uk/acts/acts2005/50009--b.htm#9

39 Daniels N, Sabin J. Limits to healthcare: fair procedures, democratic deliberation, and the legitimacy problem for insurers. *Phil & Pub Affairs.* 1997; **26**(4): 303–50.

40 Singer PA, Martin DK, Giacomini M, Purdy L. Priority setting for new technologies in medicine: qualitative case study. *BMJ.* 2000; **321**(7272): 1316–18.

Chapter 12

Final thoughts: conclusions and endnotes

Deborah Bowman and John Spicer

> Out of damp and gloomy days, out of solitude, out of loveless words directed at us, conclusions grow up in us like fungus: one morning they are there, we know not how, and they gaze upon us, morose and grey. Woe to the thinker who is not the gardener but only the soil of the plants that grow in him.[1]
>
> Friedrich Nietzsche

This book emerges from some rather scholarly fastnesses into a world of rapidly changing primary care, although those within the fastnesses are well connected with the outside world. That primary care is so described is self-evident in the UK, but it is also so in other areas of the developed world. In fact, primary care as practised in the UK is in the process of being exported to many parts of the rest of the world too. Perhaps that is indicative of its quality.

It might be inferred that we are proposing that the ethical issues predominantly affecting primary care are concerned with autonomy, error, trust, the elderly, evidence, teamworking, self-care, rights, virtue and personal faults. Such an inference would be understandable but inaccurate. The selection of issues has been driven, as stated in the introduction, by the diversity of interests and skills of the contributors. There are many other areas of content that might exercise the mind of an interested observer of the ethics of primary care. Several of these have been present in ghostly ways behind the texts of the chapters, if occasionally mentioned overtly. So the first items in the ethical crystal ball to require a passing reference are those ghosts.

Issues of resource allocation are, as in all healthcare arenas, impossible to avoid. At the time of writing, legal judgments are potentially succeeding in opening up treatments of unproven value to desperate patients by right and are creating confusion as to how treatments should be allocated.[2] The NHS, despite unparalleled investment, is rapidly reducing costs in some areas because of cash flow problems and a further shift of care from secondary to primary is proposed by government.[3] This is not the place to embark on another ethical analysis of distributive justice, but it inevitably needs to be stated that each of these facts will require ethical consideration in primary care. And what will drive that process is the political decision to return and enlarge the resource decision-making to primary care practitioners through the medium of practice-based commissioning (PBC). The authors offer no publishable view of PBC other than to advise that those professionals who find themselves making resource allocation decisions should be aware of both the ethics and the law of distributive justice, and also of notions of equity. Such was not always obviously the case in previous systems in the UK where primary care clinicians engaged in resource decision-making.

The second ghost is the place of research. The role of empiricism in ethics has been the subject of much comment[4] and our intention is not to revisit a meta-ethical debate. It is more to suggest that research into or about the ethical terrain in primary care would be of inestimable value for the future. The traditional model of ethical analysis is philosophical and reasoned. In applied ethics the methods of, for example, sociological research, have added to knowledge about how moral theory is actually interpreted and used. We know little about how clinicians in primary care derive their moral professional behaviours and why, and perhaps we should. It seems sensible to assume that those behaviours, and the moral positions that inform them, are mediated in primary care by the longstanding clinician to patient relationship, but is it actually thus? Similarly, comments made in some of the chapters on the context of the patient in his or her own milieu and how this might affect the ethics of their care are essentially derived from principle rather than the product of a framework of observation. Perhaps they should be similarly enhanced by empirical study.

The third ghost is demographic. Primary care is not immune from the population changes that Western countries are currently experiencing and arguably the most relevant is the increasing proportion of older, and dependent, people. While this will have resource implications, there will also be other issues to consider. Ethics for the care of the elderly is not a formal subject hitherto discussed at length, and has been discussed from only one point of view in this book, but it will no doubt form an increasingly important area of debate in years to come as the elderly population becomes relatively larger.

So, let us move from the spectral to the concrete and offer some crystal ball-gazing in the areas that have been addressed. What might be their future in the 21st century? We offer these from the perspective of reflection on the completion of this book, having considered the themes at length, and accept full responsibility for their provenance.

Issues of personal autonomy have been extensively considered. Each chapter has referred to respect for autonomous decision-making. Our position, derived as it is from our roles as ethicists, educators and clinicians is that the traditional Anglo-American view of personal autonomy is shifting. The familiar ethical terrain describes the principle of autonomy as pre-eminent and absolute, but the lesson from primary care is that it is not always so, nor perhaps should it always be so. It is diffused by the context of its expression, by its co-ownership with significant others and the uncertainty of events. So an ostensibly autonomous decision by a patient needs to be considered by clinicians in relation to others and the risks and possible benefits it engenders. The seductive risks of simplification are particularly potent but nonetheless unhelpful when considering primary care.

One of those others is, of course, the clinician him or herself. How might he or she affect the autonomous decision? Does a long-standing relationship with a patient, as provided in primary care, bring about a patient decision closer to that which the clinician might wish for, or not? Our suspicion is that it might be so – a suspicion crying out for empirical work – but if it is truly so, how is it to be evaluated? Furthermore, how will clinicians learn to bear both the privileges and responsibilities that arise from such a construction of autonomy as shaped by the longitudinal therapeutic relationship?

The long-standing relationship is a measure of continuity, generally held to be a good thing in itself, but it is conceivable that familiarity as an expression of continuity of care may indeed breed a less autonomous decision. Where the border between an adjusted or augmented autonomous decision and a coerced decision lies will be an area of fruitful argument in the future. Put simply, does familiarity breed consent?

The position of the clinician in relation to the professional behaviour of his or her colleagues has been a recurring theme. Must it, for example, not stray (too) far from others' behaviour? To put it differently, should clinical guidelines utterly constrain clinical decision-making? As one of the authors in this book has observed, it can be considerably more complex to bring GPs to observe guidelines and protocols than secondary care doctors. Is this necessarily a bad thing or may it work to patients' advantage on occasions? After all, one of the roles of any primary care clinician is to advocate for their patients and potentially that may involve crossing a guideline boundary. Would the primary care 'boids' discussed in Chapter 8 gain more for their patients (and themselves) by flocking or dispersing?

We suspect that a brisk or dubious attitude to clinical guidelines may benefit individual patients more where the role of clinical judgement can be allied to knowledge of protocols essentially based on population measures. Although clinical guidelines are proliferating, and arguably render practice more straightforward, the best interests of patients may be better served by adopting a healthy but informed disrespect. The ethic underlying this approach may be at variance with evolving UK common law, but that is no reason why it is wrong. And, as Brazier has observed, guidelines will keep medical lawyers busy with patient-led litigation,[5] a conclusion that leads us to resist a tempting observation about work created by diabolic entities for those with unoccupied hands.

Finally, we wish to reinforce the theme of uncertainty that has revealed itself explicitly throughout this book. The advent of a utilitarian philosophy in the 19th century for the first time looked to the future as the source of moral value. Put briefly, what was moral was that which brought about the best consequences for all. Healthcare, it is submitted, has vigorously engaged with utilitarian theory in recent years and nowhere more obviously than in the area of evidence-based care. However, the connection between the future (the apparent denominator of utilitarian judgment) and the past (the numerator) is straddled by an uncertain causation. The practice nurse and GP who between them administer the vaccination of a child cannot *know* that the vaccination will benefit, or harm, that particular child. They can make a reasonable guess based on population studies, which themselves guess at causation, but that, it seems, is all they can do. Uncertainty, like poverty, appears to be a constant and perhaps under-discussed phenomenon in healthcare, particularly primary healthcare. And yet it is the lens through which the daily work of primary care practitioners must surely be viewed.

Similarly, the health visitor considering whether to refer a child to child protection services cannot *know* whether such a referral will ultimately turn out to be in the long-term interests of the child. He or she can only suspect and hope that it will. Both those judgments are utilitarian but uncertain. And as such the uncertainty clouds the ethics of the action. It is a fact more noticeably observed in primary care than secondary and it permeates the clinical ethics.

So if there are three themes that this book has considered overtly and three themes that it has considered covertly, where might the reader seek further enlightenment? There are bodies of literature on resource allocation, empirical research in ethics and uncertainty. Research using these terms as key words or phrases will reap rich and voluminous papers, monographs and books sufficient to occupy the interested reader for a long time. However, we would suggest that a further way in which enlightenment may productively be sought is by making time for that over-used term, and perhaps under-valued concept, reflection. The primary care professional who is able to make space to grapple with these infinitely challenging ethical ghosts is more likely to find him or herself discomforted than enlightened perhaps. However, the discomforting nature of ethics is the intellectual equivalent of the trite mantra of aerobics instructors in the 1980s – 'no pain, no gain'. These are not issues that are susceptible to easy, neat and swift answers. A conclusion that claimed otherwise would do its readers and, ultimately, patients a great disservice. These are issues that warrant careful and measured attention – the sort of attention that depends on that rare commodity for busy primary care professionals – time. If primary healthcare teams can eke out time to consider and discuss these complex questions, we will be content. Thus, if this book provides a starting point for, or material to inform, these reflective discussions, we will be delighted.

Such reflections, which may be case-based or more general, are part of an ethical process that has value in and of itself. While concentration on the outcome of discussion and reflection is more immediately attractive, perhaps, we suggest that the process described is part of the ascription of right and wrong, of ethical or unethical, of professional or unprofessional.

References

1 Nietzsche F. *Daybreak: thoughts on the prejudices.* Cambridge Texts in the History of Philosophy. Cambridge: Cambridge University Press; 1997.
2 *R (Rogers) v Swindon NHS Primary Care Trust* [2006] EWCA Civ 392.
3 Department of Health. *Our Health, Our Care, Our Say: a new direction for community services.* Cmnd Paper 6737. London: The Stationery Office; 2006.
4 Hope T. Empirical medical ethics. *J Med Ethics.* 1999; **25**(June): 219–20; Borry P, Schotsmans P, Dierickx K. Empirical research in bioethical journals. A quantitative analysis. *J Med Ethics.* 2006; **32**(April): 240–5.
5 Brazier M. Times of change. *Med Law Rev.* 2005; **13**(Spring): 1–16.

Index